TEACHING NURSING: A SELF-INSTRUCTIONAL HANDBOOK

Teaching Nursing
A Self-Instructional Handbook

CHRISTINE EWAN *PhD*
and RUTH WHITE *R.N., EdD*

CROOM HELM
London • New York • Sydney

© 1984 Christine Ewan and Ruth White
Croom Helm Ltd, Provident House, Burrell Row,
Beckenham, Kent, BR3 1AT
Croom Helm Australia, 44-50 Waterloo Road,
North Ryde, 2113, New South Wales
Reprinted 1986 and 1987

British Library Cataloguing in Publication Data

Ewan, Christine E.
   Teaching nursing.
   1. Nursing—Study and teaching
   I. Title II. White, Ruth
   610.73'07'11   RT73
   ISBN 0-7099-0936-5

Published in the USA by
Croom Helm
in association with Methuen, Inc.
29 West 35th Street
New York, NY 10001

Library of Congress Cataloging-in-Publication Data

Ewan, Christine E.
   Teaching nursing.

   Includes index.
   1. Nursing—Study and teaching. 2. Nursing—
Study and teaching—Problems, exercises, etc.
I. White, Ruth, 1926- . II. Title.
RT90.E93   1984   610.73'07   84-16980
ISBN 0-7099-0936-5 (pbk.)

Printed and bound in Great Britain by
Biddles Ltd, Guildford and King's Lynn

CONTENTS

List of Tables & Figures
Introduction

TABLES AND FIGURES

INTRODUCTION

Nursing education is facing a challenging period as the roles of the nurse and the training required to fulfil those roles undergo critical reexamination. This book has been written to provide a personal guide to the new educational practices, and to some of the more traditional approaches, for teachers who will be involved in educating nurses for the future.

The first chapter reviews trends which have emerged in nursing education to equip nurses for their changed roles and responsibilities in the changed environment of modern health services, the second chapter examines the techniques which can be used by teachers or by curriculum planners to determine relevant content for nursing courses and chapter three provides an overview of the learning process presented as the basis for decisions about teaching. Chapter four offers guidelines for the choice and design of teaching methods which accommodate both the content and objectives of courses and the learning processes of students. Active student involvement, students' acceptance of responsibility for their own learning, and the development of professional skills and approaches are emphasised. Chapter five discusses specific topics in nursing education which require innovative approaches to teaching and learning and provides some examples of applications of the processes and methods discussed in preceding chapters, while the sixth chapter expands on those methods and processes with particular reference to the use of learning resources. Chapters seven and eight address the purposes and methods for assessment of student performance and evaluation of courses and teaching. Once again emphasis is placed upon the development among students, of professional skills in establishing criteria, using feedback constructively, and evaluating their own and their colleagues' performances.

In keeping with our overall philosophy of the necessity for active involvement of learners in relevant activity, most of the chapters in this book are self-instructional in the sense that they invite the reader to undertake activities which involve analysis of personal teaching conditions and practices, and which encourage the design or development of approaches to specific teaching objectives or problems. Feedback to each of these activities forms the bulk of the text and it is possible to read the book without undertaking the activities. The decision is yours, however we recommend the activities to you because they have been chosen from questions most commonly asked by teachers attending our courses and the chances are that many represent questions that you have also asked yourself in the course of your teaching. Attention to the activities will ensure that your personal questions are called to mind and that you are able to apply the content of the feedback to specific aspects of your situation rather than attempting to remember it as general information.

We have attempted to keep the content of the book relatively jargon-free, readable and practical, sometimes at the expense of doing systematic justice to educational theory. We hope that the theorists among our readers will forgive this decision and use the references provided for their specific needs and interests. We also hope that readers with little formal training in educational theory and practice will use this book as an introduction and be stimulated to follow up areas of personal interest among the material offered as references.

Finally, we would both wish to acknowledge, with warm appreciation of her skills and gratitude for her unfailing patience, the contribution to this text of Mrs. Helen Fodor. The preparation of the manuscript would not have been accomplished without her willing participation in typing, checking and attending to the myriad of details involved.

Christine Ewan
Ruth White

TEACHING NURSING: A SELF-INSTRUCTIONAL HANDBOOK

Chapter 1

TRENDS IN NURSE EDUCATION

INTRODUCTION

Throughout the following chapters in this book
you will find many opportunities for testing your
knowledge about teaching students to nurse, trying
out your own ideas, and discovering their worth,
and for increasing your skills in assisting
students to learn.

In this introductory chapter, the intention is
to outline some of the forces and trends
influencing nurse education today. There are many
trends at present which are directing what we teach
and the way we teach it. Some of these trends have
had (and are having) an influence on the way
nursing is conceptualised as a subject for study.
Others are affecting the way nursing is practised.
In many schools of nursing, curricula are being
developed which reflect these major trends and
consequently the substance and methods of teaching
are changing.

FORCES AFFECTING NURSE EDUCATION

Not surprisingly, most of the forces impinging
upon general education also pose important
questions for nurse education. Forces such as the
explosion of knowledge and the increasing
sophistication of technology affect all systems of
education in the eighties. On a social level,
forces of political, economic and socio-cultural
dimensions are not exclusive to the nation's
general education but evoke responses from
sub-systems of education of which nurse

1

education is one. Within nurse education itself forces in the form of movements (such as professionalisation, specialisation) exert their impact and demand a response. Important also, as a force, is the strength of the women's movement and the effect that movement has had on raising awareness of the general population (and nurses in particular) of the legitimacy of human rights in a broad sense and patient's rights in the context of health and welfare.

Knowledge explosion

'An information bomb' Toffler (1981) declares, 'is exploding in our midst, showering us with a shrapnel of images and drastically changing the way each of us perceives and acts upon our private world'. We can now study phenomena hitherto impossible to explore because they were too ephemeral, too distant, too miniscule or too complex to detect with conventional equipment. It is now possible not only to marvel at the explanations of phenomena but to experience humankind's advances by, for example, walking in space, retrieving vast displays of information, 'seeing' inside the human body at fractional depths and angles through integrated computerised imaging. The information obtained has made the generalist obsolete; the specialist supreme.

Technological expansion

Scarcely a sphere of society, let alone education, has been unaffected by the advances in technology. The tools of education now include video and computer. The organisation of programs is no longer constrained by size of class or presence of teacher since mass communication by satellite is a reality.

The ease with which children have access to, and manage video and computer games, has direct impact on our ideas of how students learn. Now that it is possible to link numbers of institutions to access results from various research studies and to store, analyse and retrieve data, the implications for educational research have yet to be realised. Exploiting the new technologies for education, industry and the professions is a required skill for educational planners and teachers.

Sophisticated technology has been increasing its impact on the health care system, not only in the availability of a range of diagnostic tests but, also, in increasing the safety, validity and reliability of test results. The variety of therapies at the disposal of health professionals has increased. Again, the implications of the new technologies are as wide ranging for medical and health services research as they are for education. On the one hand producing exhilarating hope for previously untreatable sufferers and on the other, despair and despondency for ethical decision-makers forced to choose among many needy individuals for the limited and astronomically expensive high technological resources.

Anticipating the modern dilemma Celebreeze (1966) indicated the central issue almost twenty years ago:

'The question that education has not yet answered is the question that technology poses for our entire society - the question of its mastery for human aims and human uses rather than for its own sake.'

Specialisation

As a response to the increase in knowledge and technology, specialisation in a specific area of knowledge, expertise or technique has become a force within many occupations and professions. An obvious corollary is the lengthening of the hierarchy within professions and the consequent demarcation, splintering and fragmentation of the service provided.

As a driving force in health care, specialisation has splintered broad areas of treatment into smaller specialties and the rate of technological change has involved the specialist in an endless study and pursuit of the most up-to-date advances. With such a concentration of effort on smaller and smaller specialisations the communication of specialists across different disciplines becomes almost impossible. Even if time and inclination allowed, the need to master the technical language, in order to challenge the monopoly of esoteric knowledge, poses a deterrent for the most courageous inter-disciplinarian.

3

Professionalisation

Swayed by issues of the status of the expert the power of superior knowledge and technology and the rewards that accompany specialist expertise, professionalisation has been a powerful force affecting most of the labour force. Education and health care have not escaped and nurse education has a history of progressive rise on the professional ladder. A criticism often made of a profession aiming for recognition of its role in society vis-a-vis the service it provides is the issue of status seeking. Furthermore, attempts to improve the education foundation of a profession and the qualification of its members is often labelled with the accusation of credentialism.

A powerful force in challenging both the legitimacy of the expert and the status of professional eminence is the current popularity of self-help groups, community action, alternative education and health movement, and environmental lobbies, the latter on a world-wide scale.

Political and economical forces

Recent government decisions in many countries threaten the accessibility to higher education of many thousands of young people who might have hoped to enter. The possible closure of some universities and amalgamations of educational institutions is a fact of educational administrative life. With limited resources of finance and equipment and also of personnel, the fear of reduced opportunities to carry out research is a major threat to educational and health research.

It would be hard to find a country whose health system was not affected by current political and economic forces. The macro-structure in which nursing education is planned is therefore subject to political decisions about its future expansion or contraction, economic strictures on the provision of resources and materials and the social responsibility to take a stand on many world issues such as nuclear involvement, population control or the environment.

In the western world there are forces impinging upon nursing education arising directly out of the health care system itself. For example, the contentious arguments about the advantages and disadvantages of high technology; the claim that redress of balance between acute and preventive care is overdue; and the often painful decisions required in bio-ethics are areas of concern indicating the complexities in the current scene.

The developing world's concern with day to day demands for the essentials of food, water, shelter and safety put the previous problems into a perspective often unappreciable by many who will use this book.

Social and cultural forces

In general education the effect of the movements such as human rights and conservation (to name a few) have acted as a force for change.

A considerable literature exists on the access of women to higher education, the success rate of mature aged women in higher degree study and the pressures affecting academic visibility, promotion and publications. Symptomatic of the force of the women's movement is the 1984 title of the World Yearbook of Education - Women and Education. This publication shows how the social, political and economic content of education influences the lives and roles of women and also how education can be used by women to change their lives for the better (Acker et al. 1984).

TRENDS IN NURSE EDUCATION - RESPONSE TO THE FORCES

Why mention these macro-structure factors when the text is set in the micro-structure of the day to day decisions about how to teach nursing and how students best learn to nurse? Yet these issues have relevance for nurse educators whatever our national setting and background because we express, as individuals, our values and beliefs on these major concerns, to students and to colleagues. As teachers, these values and beliefs are often on show to students in 'off guard' moments and our teaching cannot but reflect the importance to us of the forces in which the society around us exists. To colleagues, the decisions we make about content in a course, its sequencing and its presentation to students, are often indications of the underlying attitudes and values we hold about learning and achievement in society; about co-operation or competition; about control or constraint.

There can be little argument with the fact that awareness of national or of world forces leads us to think through the relevance of what is taught to students and to consider with more understanding the context in which students will practise on graduation.

Knowledge and Nursing

Identifying nursing knowledge from the vast stores of information available is an important trend in response to the explosion of knowledge. The trend is recognisable by the numbers of articles and texts documenting the progress of theory development (Stevens, 1979; Chinn & Jacobs, 1983) research into nursing practice and education [Hill et al., 1980; Journal of Nursing Education (whole issue) Oct. 1982; Davis 1983]) the rise of conceptual systems to explain nursing (Fawcett, 1980) and the emergence of a nursing science (Stainton, 1982).

The effect of the trend is to identify a distinct focus for nursing. There are various ways of expressing the focus, but in general, the basic concepts of person, health, nursing and environment are included. These concepts form the foundation or framework for the development of theories of nursing and provide a source of nursing knowledge. It goes without saying that the perception nurses have of the basic concepts is influential in determining how knowledge will be selected, taught and transferred to practice.

> 'The importance of the trend towards using conceptual systems of nursing as guides for education, practice and research activities of nurses cannot be over-emphasized. Since these models provide a distinct focus for nursing, they can increase nurses' confidence that what they are doing is nursing, not medicine, not social work, nor the function of any other health profession.'
> (Fawcett, 1980 p.312).)

Later in this book (Chapter 2) a number of methods for selecting content for teaching are discussed. At the level of deciding what to teach within a course, you are also identifying nursing knowledge. The trend we are discussing at the moment is set on a broader professional level. It is not surprising, therefore, to find statements indicating the direction of the trend, such as:

> '... the phenomenal field of nursing (is) not **nursing** , but the health seeking behaviours of humans, their responses to illness and their coping behaviours in attaining or maintaining health.'
> (Stainton, 1982 p. 27)

and

> '... any study concerned with dimensions of clients' health has potential for building a requisite knowledge base.'
> (Fawcett, 1980 p. 313)

Technology and Nursing

Multi-skilling is a trend discussed by Brewer (1983) as a response to the expansion of technology and technological change. Preparing nurses for practice in **the age of discontinuity** requires an education to maintain relevancy in a rapidly changing technological environment, to use personal and therapeutic skills of 'touch' to communicate with unconscious patients, and to apply technical, co-ordinating and monitoring skills.

The accelerated trend for nursing education to include ethical decision-making in the nursing program is directly related to the dilemmas raised by technological change. Finding a balance between care and cure; protecting the humanity as well as the health of a patient; assisting patients to clarify their values and beliefs are issues discussed by Benoliel (1983). Levine (1980) reminds us of the potential of machines to de-personalise nurses and patients and the need to protect each other from the indifference of the machine.

Strategies for identifying and responding to complex moral problems, such as ethical inquiry and analyses are included in Chapter 5 together with suggested methods for teaching students to think through the ethical components of a problem in patient care.

The trend towards developing the caring nature of nursing with particular regard to the technological pressures on people at work, leisure or when incapacitated or ill, is expressed by Carper (1978):

'Nursing as a genuinely caring enterprise, firmly anchored in respect for the dignity and worth of the person being cared for, is perhaps the source for mitigating the dehumanising tendencies inherent in today's highly institutionalised and technologically oriented health care delivery.'

An important trend influencing the care of children, particularly, in developing countries, is the application of appropriate technology to solve problems on a community as well as on individual scale. The simple method of administration of oral rehydration has demonstrated the dramatic curative effect of timely, low cost, highly relevant, easily prepared and administrated technology. Nurse educators have an important role to play in indicating the importance of 'low' technology, as well as the visible 'high' technology.

Politics, power, professionalism and primary health care nursing

Primary health care, a strong trend in the last decades of this century, draws attention to the rights of persons to health care. Considerably more than that in its intent, primary health care changes the relationships between professional power and the population.

As a response to the political and economic forces responsible for the distribution of wealth and resources, primary health care is a powerful trend towards integration of services in the interests of the provision of basic human needs.

For nurse education the trend is important as it is necessary to prepare nurses to discover different life styles and different communities. Educational programs in nursing with a strong hospital orientation require review to widen the experiences of students. Bringing people into decision-making requires skills which need to be fostered through practice. For the student who learns that nursing is predominantly a one-to-one relationship dealing with community groups may be outside 'nursing'. Primary health care involves the nurse in actively assisting people and groups in self-determination and in making decisions based on their own goals.

Primary health care is also a response to the

social and cultural forces impinging on the right
of individuals. Health personnel no longer hold the
monopoly of knowledge. In fact unless the community
assists the professional to understand what primary
health care means in their particular context, a
barrier between them will exist and knowledge will
not be shared.

> 'In the primary health care approach, care
> actions cannot be dissociated from social
> actions since everything that affects
> health has a social element. This means
> re-emphasising the social dimension of nursing
> and recognising its social influence as well
> as the link with other networks of health and
> social action.'
> (Colliere, 1980, p. 169)

Ways of knowing
        The potential for several interesting debates
exist in nursing: The pressure toward professionalisation and recognition of nursing as a
discipline (Donaldson & Crowley, 1978) and the
realisation that professionalism carries with it
exclusiveness, elitism, restriction of entry and
barriers of language, style and conventions is an
ethical problem in the making.
        Another debating point is the issue of
scientific problem-solving as the preferred mode
for nursing practice. Those who support this view
do so from the conviction that problems form the
basis of practice and following the steps of
problem-solving is a rational, respected scientific
method. Those who find this stance unsatisfactory,
do so from two main themes. One holds that
intuition should not be discounted as a nursing
skill and that intuitive reasoning should not be
devalued and omitted from nursing practice. The
other claims that a limited view of problem-solving
obtains when computerised programs break down the
components of a person's problem into small bits.
At that point appreciation of the whole person is
almost a lost perspective.The trend to analyse
critically the divergent views expressed in nursing
is a healthy sign of colleagueship and security in
the ability to admit a different view.
        The trend for curricula in nurse education to
be integrated in design and based on a conceptual

framework where the whole person is considered in interaction with the environment is directly related to the forces which threaten the holistic nature of humankind. Specialism, we noticed, resulted in the separation of knowledge and of professionals into smaller and smaller compartments. Holism, on the other hand, operates from the opposite view and assists health workers to perceive not separate components of a person, but the whole person in that person's context. The nature of nursing has been described from that basis:

'..... nursing studies the wholeness or health of humans, recognising that humans are in continuous interaction with their environment.' (Donaldson and Crowley, 1978, p. 119)

That is why the 'ways of knowing' in nursing include aesthetic, ethical, personal knowledge as well as empirical knowledge. (Carper, 1978).

Students, teachers and the nursing program

How is it possible to address all of the issues that ebb and flow in and around nursing problems? When forces of such magnitude as the human need for survival and the advancing sophistication of technology encroaches upon decisions about what to teach and how students will learn to nurse, the individual teacher in a classroom or in the field (clinical or community) seems powerless to contribute to the direction nursing education will take. In fact, reversing the order of learning rather than teaching, as the trend suggests, thus putting the responsibility of their continuing learning on to students, may appear to be a retreat from facing a very real problem in schools of nursing - that is - how to manage the demands of a full curriculum in the time available.

It would seem that where programs have centred on the students' need to be active learners, to react to ideas, to respond to critical questions and to apply knowledge to individual patient's problems,the accent has been on 'getting out of the students' way' so that they can learn in their own way. Interestingly, the resulting nursing practice often reflects these attitudes. Rather than hemming

10

the patient in with routines and rituals and uniform requirements for recovery, the idea of letting patients set the pace for their progress according to individual needs, has evolved.

Later in this book (Chapter 4) the ways of assisting students to learn with or without the teacher will be outlined and the emphasis on learning rather than teaching is shown to have justification in nurse education. In fact, this book itself is a learning rather than a teaching resource turning over to the reader guidelines, ideas and strategies for the teacher to assess, critique and decide on their use.

Curriculum

Across the nursing world a common trend is the challenge of traditional nursing programs. In these traditional programs the study of diseases is the basis of the curriculum and the recall of aetiology, signs and symptoms, treatment, prognosis and nursing care is evidence of completion of the course, as reflected in a successful pass in examination papers, and the termination of a rotation through all of the departments where the major diseases and conditions are treated.

Further, the trend is to claim that the curricula in the past have fastened on to parts of the person (disease, problem, body system) thus directing students to learn according to discrete components and to practise nursing in separate departments often with dissimilar objectives within the same institution.

Faced with the growing pressure to identify 'what is nursing', the trend in many countries is to claim that the whole person is the focus of nursing. That both 'whole' and 'health' derive from the same root 'hal' is confirmation for many nurses that the whole person and health are valid concepts thereby strengthening each other providing a rationale for the current concern about health as well as illness.

A sweeping trend at present is to think in terms of an holistic curriculum. The basic concepts are generally, man, health, nursing and environment; the aim is to consider the person as a total human being within a number of contexts. This encourages the integration of subjects and the blurring of traditional discipline boundaries.

11

Nurses in such a program, it is claimed, learn to practise care for the 'whole person'.

Some nurses believe that what is distinctive about nursing therefore, is that nurses take their priorities directly from the patient/client (whole person) rather than from the treatment regime, the disease process, or the technological prescription. This puts an emphasis on phenomena which have always claimed the attention of nurses during their span of contact with patients and which, until recently, have not been studied nor investigated for their importance in patient comfort, care or cure. Examples of these phenomena are - emergence of pain, restlessness, discomfort, dependence.

On broader curriculum lines, learning about the whole person in context would be approached from an organizing theme of life phases, or age continuum, or the continuum of contexts - individual-family-society. Proponents of this curriculum model believe that in addition to the one-to-one interaction emphasis implied in the whole patient (holistic) curriculum there is a need to practise with different skills in relation to communities. In fact there is a strong trend to challenge nursing programs which do not address the principles of primary health care and which do not show the relevance of their teaching and practice to the commitment of the International Council of Nurses to the World Health Organization's plan for 'health for all by the year 2000'. Management of whole communities or groups as well as the care of whole persons is a current challenge for inclusion in nursing programs.

Toward a discipline of nursing

Teachers are often in a dilemma when confronted with the question of whether to teach for current practice or whether to make students more aware of the trends in nursing knowledge with which they will have to deal later as graduates. The issue seems to be whether teachers consider nursing as a subject worthy of serious study and scholarship, (a discipline in its own right) or a field of professional practice or both of these. There are excellent discussions on the progress of nursing as a discipline which illuminate this issue for nurse educators and nurse clinicians alike. (Stevens, 1979; Donaldson and Crowley, 1978).

The issue of relevance of the curriculum to current practice is important, but equally important is the option of assisting students to think towards the future, extending their ideas about human welfare, and their own potential for effectiveness in health care. In a world of such rapid change as we are experiencing, the 'need for preparation for change' is a cliche - overworn and out of date. A future orientation seems unarguable. Moreover, there are many sources of assistance available now to nurse teachers seeking to revitalize their teaching, or to study curriculum development. A growing literature, and the existence of professional groups interested in educational development both within nursing and across the disciplines is evidence of increasing activity in the field of health professional education generally and nurse education in particular.

Research in nurse education
    Research in nurse education has developed rapidly from studies of the role of teachers, characteristics of students, attrition and retention rates and comparative forms of assessing the competencies of students, to tackle the more nebulous areas of identifying key concepts for the practice of nursing, integrating theory and practice, skills of clinical teaching, and nursing curriculum and program evaluation (Infante 1975; Allen, 1977). Particularly interesting to nurse teachers, because of the potential for adding to nursing knowledge, are the studies where nurses have departed from the pattern set by other disciplines and have used a model of inquiry more appropriate to the discipline of nursing itself (Davis, 1983; Morse, 1983; Creighton, 1983).

Theory development in Nursing
    Even as recently as the last decade there has been a vast increase in theory development in nursing and in the formulation of the conceptual base of nursing practice [Chinn and Jacobs (1983) give an overview of the work of seventeen current theorists]. There may not be agreement about the elements of the concepts or the substance of the theories; in fact, as it is claimed, there is much theorising and few theories. Nevertheless, the

activity in the profession in many countries is a major force in directing attention towards the complex task of identifying what constitutes appropriate nursing knowledge relevant to practice in the twenty first century.

CONCLUSION - TOWARDS THE FUTURE

Because curriculum development can be a powerful force in directing the future of any professional field, the recognition of its place in nursing has been a step of the greatest importance bringing with it the need to increase the curriculum planning and development skills of teachers. With the entry of nursing education into higher education in many countries has come the opportunity to develop curricula and to design teaching occasions and learning contexts appropriate to the people needing health care and to the needs of adult students who will practise nursing with a broader and deeper theoretical base than has been possible in student/apprenticeship programs.

There has probably never been a more exciting time in which to develop programs, to help nurses to learn, and to make changes in the way nursing is practised. The direction of those changes is conditional on the extent to which nurses can examine the current forces and trends and assess the most useful ways in which nursing can respond for the betterment of the care of patients, the education of professionally and socially responsible students, and the effectiveness of health care generally.

Chapter 2

DECIDING WHAT TO TEACH

Whatever your role in teaching students to
nurse you will have some responsibility in deciding
what you will teach. Even though you may be given a
prescribed area or topic, with little room to
manoeuvre, the emphasis you choose to give to
components of the topic will quickly indicate to
students your preferences, values and goals.

The purpose of this chapter is to identify
ways of determining relevant content for teaching
nursing. Relevant for what and for whom are issues
which will be threaded through the activities and
discussion as they are basic to the decisions
teachers make in choosing content.

Although it is true that deciding what to
teach is largely a question for the total
curriculum, it is not the intention in this text to
discuss curriculum design and structure in detail.
There are several informative texts on curriculum
planning in nurse education (e.g. Bevis, 1973;
Conley, 1973; Heath, 1982) and many in general
education (Taba, 1962; Warwick, 1973; Stenhouse,
1975; Kerr, 1976) where curriculum issues may be
read in detail. On the other hand there are few
resources to assist the teacher in classroom,
clinical or community teaching (be they trained
teachers or clinicians who teach only occasionally)
to decide what should be taught in relation to a
particular group or class of students in the
context of health services.

In using the format of activities, feedback
and discussion, it is hoped that day to day issues
and problems in selecting relevant teaching
material will surface and that the suggested
techniques for dealing with determining content
will prove useful.

When you finish this chapter **you should be able to recognise the basis of the decisions you make in choosing what to teach and be able to use a variety of techniques for determining content for assisting students to learn to nurse.**

Why is deciding what to teach such a problem in nursing? If we look at what students think they are learning there is little doubt that it is a major issue. For example Melia (1982) found that students' descriptions of nursing can be summed up in three ways:

Real nursing   - i.e. technically oriented
                                    work
Not really nursing - i.e. social care such as
                                    long stay geriatric
                                    patients
Just basic nursing - i.e. nursing care which
                                    is independent of medical
                                    prescription.

If we also look at the work that experienced R.N.s do in - say - critical care (the 'Real' nursing alluded to above) we would probably conclude with Baumann (1982) that there is a problem with the content chosen for graduate students' programs also. Baumann found that critical care nurses were competent in making rapid decisions in a given crisis, but they had difficulty in providing the theoretical basis for their decision.

What do these two studies illustrate? Perhaps all we should say at this point is that they represent the tip of the proverbial iceberg; pre- and post-registration courses alike are often subject to confusion regarding the most appropriate content to be chosen. It would be interesting to trace **how** the content for critical care nursing was chosen as well as **what** content formed the course.

Activity:
Choose an area or topic you are currently teaching, or planning to teach and make a list of what you consider your students must know. In your list underline the most important items. Find a colleague and explain your

rationale, justifying your selection of 'most important' items.

Feedback:

Naturally enough you may have found this activity irritating as it is such a fundamental question to answer and obviously there are no right or wrong answers. In explaining your rationale you may have found a few contentious issues. The point of the activity, is of course, the task of identifying the basis of your decisions about what to teach. You may have justified your list by citing the importance of clinical nursing.

For example, Miller (1975) observed deficiencies in the way students performed and concluded that content should be chosen which specifies the **correct action** to be taken, given a specific pathophysiological problem. Her rationale was that content should be determined in close relation to current practice (p.222), the first step being 'to analyze the pathophysiological problems to determine the appropriate cognitive and technical skills to be used in solving the problems and the correct actions to implement those skills. On this basis curriculum content and structure could be identified.'

Another example of using clinical problems as a basis for deciding content is found in programs built on Henderson's (1966) approach. The problems of **the activities of daily living** of individuals (sick or well) form the subject matter. Similarly, the activities of daily living are taken as the starting point by Myra Roper (1980). For both Henderson and Roper the rationale is that the 'unique function' or the primary purpose of the nurse is to assist individuals in identifying their needs and to assist them in those activities they are unable to perform themselves.

A third example comes from psychiatric nursing. Reynolds and Cormack (1982) gives as a rationale for deriving content from clinical problems the fact that teachers must know exactly **how nurses spend their time** in contact with patients in order for teaching to be relevant. He explains that because the skills of interpersonal relationships and patient teaching have such low visibility, compared with the high visibility of

17

physical care and technology, they are often not accorded a prominent place in teaching.

Lastly, Jerrett and Ross (1982) also observe the nurse in practice to decide content. They claim that although students may have direct contact with a single patient this is done within the complexities of health care and content therefore begins with **the whole situation.** Nurses and patients, their families and communities exist in a social context and observing practice therefore involves more than focusing on a one to one direct relationship of nurse and patient.

The interesting point is that although all four examples took as their starting point the question what do nurses do? - their conclusions about what the nurse should know are dissimilar.

TABLE 2.1 : BASIS FOR CONTENT DECISIONS

Focus of clini- cal observation	Content	Justification
1. Deficiencies in practice	Pathophysiol- ogical problems. Cognitive & technical skills.	Need for correct action
2. Individuals sick or well	Problems of activities of daily living. How to assist.	Unique function of nurse
3. Exactly how time is spent by nurse in contact with patients	Interpersonal interaction therapeutics	As import- ant as high visi- bility care
4. Direct care within com- plexities of health care	Whole situation of the patient	Social contact of individuals families communities
5.		

Their view of nursing (and what the nurse should be) are different, and therefore the focus of their observation is different in each case. Naturally decisions about what to teach are affected as the content column above, shows.

In order to identify how your selection of content was made it may be helpful to add the result of the activity (p. 16) to the summary on page 18 in the space allowed - '5'.

Try to condense your list of 'most important' content to a few concepts before entering your result in column 2. Then insert your rationale as derived when explaining your selection of content to your colleague. Unless you have recently been involved in a systematic observation of students' practice, (e.g. task analysis or some other technique) you probably used your own experience, background knowledge and preferences to make the selection, so column 1 will not be necessary. That leaves column 3. For our purposes, this is the most interesting.

Activity:
Consider all of the entries in columns 2 and 3 including your own. On what basis was your selection of content made? Look at column 3 again. Does your justification differ markedly from the others?

Feedback:
Possibly your justification was the use of a model of nursing. The base of your decision in that case is clear; content is derived from the theoretical support for the model. (We will discuss nursing models and conceptual frameworks later in this Chapter.)

On the other hand your justification could rest on the needs of a specialist area, e.g. neonatal intensive care. In this case the objectives and competencies to be mastered by the end of the course would be clearly and precisely stated. Alternatively, if your justification is in terms of some future role or function which you envisage your students will be called upon to

19

perform, then the basis of your decision about what to teach will be made after an exercise in future forecasting. (This technique will also be included later in the Chapter.)

Then again, in the daily bustle of a busy program, decisions about what to teach are often made, quite frankly, on the spur of the moment; from the teachers' current research work; from the dictates of an examination system; on the immediate needs of a practice or service area; or a number of other reasons based more on administrative necessity or personal convenience of the teacher than on a carefully arrived at rationale for student learning. Naturally the benefits of this approach for students, are questionable.

Summary

What can be inferred from the table? We began by asking the question - What must your students learn and why - Activity p.16. The feedback took the form of examples from the experiences of several teachers showing how they decided what was important to teach and giving their justification. Like Stevens (1979) they would subscribe to the view that nurse education is concerned with 'the translation of knowledge into professional acts.' Their starting point was the 'professional acts' that nurses perform. However, from the table above we can infer that asking 'What does the nurse do?' is not enough. We must also ask 'What kind of person (nurse) do we want?' and lastly, on the basis of the two preceding questions - 'What must the nurse know, and how will it be learned?'

We have now reached the point where a set of criteria for determining what to teach can be derived.

CRITERIA FOR DETERMINING CONTENT

Activity:
Imagine you are fortunate enough to have a long lead-time to prepare to teach your course. You also have been given a free hand to select the content. As you survey the increases in scientific knowledge, the

complexities of modern health services and
your particular group of students, what
criteria will you have in mind to help you
to select the content of your course?

Feedback:
   The first criterion is an obvious one. Because
nursing is a practical profession what is taught
must be **relevant** to practice.
   Second, because the content chosen will be the
focus of student learning, it should be consistent
with the way students will learn subject matter,
learn how to translate it into practice and learn
how to nurse. **Learning** and the **learner** make up the
third criterion.
   The third criterion may not be so obvious but
in recent years the number of nurses who are
prepared to present their values and beliefs about
nursing, man, health or community, to name only a
few elements, is increasing. The criterion for
choosing content, for them, is the **perspective** they
hold on what nursing is, and about how nursing
should be practised, taught and researched.
   You may have listed additional criteria such
as time available, accessibility of resources or
type of facilities for teaching. The latter may
include whether you will teach mainly in the classroom or in a practical setting in a hospital, or a
community.
   Those aspects are certainly important as they
can facilitate your planning or be a major
constraint on what is possible to include in a
course. Some of these aspects are dealt with in
other chapters and suggestions for alternative
teaching arrangements are given, particularly in
chapter 4. In this Chapter we will concentrate more
on the criteria that you as a teacher personally
and individually will choose in deciding what your
students will learn.

Relevance
   There is a full discussion in the next chapter
on relevance as one of the conditions for learning.
Its importance for motivating students and for
making learning meaningful is argued. In this
chapter our concern is more with relevance as a
criterion for the selection of what to teach in the

first place. Logically, decisions about relevant content lead to the organisation of learning sessions to enable students to appreciate the relevance of what they are learning to the accomplishment of a personal or professional goal.

The focus of relevance in deciding content in this text is believed to be the needs of students influenced by:

. their prior knowledge of the subject
. their background and experience
. their aspirations and the context in which they hope to realise them
. the activities (professional nursing acts) they will have to perform as graduates in current practice
. their perception of future tasks and activities in changing health services
. the roles they will enact in the performance of those activities
. the context in which they will function.

A criticism often made of this approach is that patients and their needs and problems should be the primary focus of decisions about content of nursing courses. However, while such a view has validity (especially when considered in its broadest sense to include planning and administration of health services to meet these needs) a backward glance at Table 2.1, reminds us that the way patients' needs and problems are perceived can result in a widely dissimilar array of content, and consequently the possibility of irrelevant learning for students.

If you have ever had the misfortune of being locked into a course where the teacher's choice of content was really meant for some other group of students, or was chosen because of a personal preference – or bias – but had no link with its translation into practice, you will have experienced a very interesting and possibly expert course of lectures, but you would have been left wondering about your ability to perform competently as a result of your experience.

Another criticism is that students' education will be limited to their own personal development and to 'doing a job.' The fear of some is that the broader aspects of education and the scientific basis of what they are doing will be omitted. One would have to agree that this is a reasonable criticism and could be true of some programs where nursing is conceptualised and practised as a set of tasks. There is a wealth of work being produced at present to show that nursing itself is evolving towards a discipline of study (Donaldson & Crowley, 1978; Stevens, 1979; Fawcett, 1980; Adam, 1983, and many more) and is educative in the truest sense as well as being a preparation for competent performance.

There are several techniques for finding out what students will be required to do as graduates in the workforce. Some of these techniques are major projects and involve time, money and research expertise and are appropriately carried out as part of the planning of an entire curriculum. For example:

(1) Observational techniques for studying current practice by direct observation, video or audio-tape.
Task analysis.
Situation analysis.

(2) Forecasting techniques for predicting possible future practice priorities.
Delphi probe. (Helmer, 1967)

(3) Surveying discrete work situations.
Job description.

To summarize what has been said about the criterion of relevance, the questions to ask and the techniques for answering them are:

Criterion	Questions	Techniques
Relevance	What does the nurse do?	Task analysis
		Job description
	What is the context?	Situation analysis
	What could be expected in the future?	Future forecasting

Learning and the Learner

The criterion for selecting content based on the student as a learner has not always been recognised in nursing courses. Rather, the selection has been made more often on the basis of its usefulness for immediate practice without consideration of the underlying understanding and principles which would enable its transfer to other situations.

Content for learning implies different goals for the learner than content for action. For example if you want students to learn by means of their clinical experience placements your expectations of what is to be learned need to be stated as distinct from what you expect the students to do. Bauman's (1982) survey on intensive care nurses' decision-making discussed earlier illustrates this point. Directing the nurse to give a rationale for the decisions made during crisis care and to trace the sequence of components in decision making for individual patients, so that future decisions would be based on a recognisable rationale has vastly different learning implications than simply instructing the nurse to list the decisions made during emergencies.

Applying the criterion of the learner to the selection of content throws the spotlight on the learner's responsibility for meeting her/his own learning needs. This requires skill on the part of the learner; a process to be developed so that dependence on the teacher is reduced. The content of a course is therefore not comprised of subject matter only, but process and environment as well.

Another important consideration is the match between the method of learning advocated in the course and the method chosen for nursing practice. Learning and practice are so intertwined that it is important that in choosing content the method of learning does not conflict with the method advocated for practice. For example, if problem solving is decided to be the relevant learning mode for a particular course, then nursing process would be an appropriate choice for practice so that students would find that learning and practice complemented each other.

Again if a certain group of competencies have been identified as the goal for the learner then the choice of content should be guided by the

24

necessary knowledge, skill and attitudes to reach competency. An integrated set of content is required in order that the application to practice is effected and the student is assisted in making further transfer to other situations. Stevens (1979) points to the inconsistencies which plague nursing whereby, for example, a discrete subject or disease centred curriculum is taught to students who will use a problem solving method in practice.

To summarise the criterion of Learning and the Learner, the following questions and techniques are included:

Criterion	Questions	Techniques
Learning and the Learner	What must the nurse know?	Objectives
		Competencies
	How will the knowledge be used?	Problem-solving

Perspective on Nursing

By now you will probably agree that choosing content for the transmission of nursing knowledge and its translation into practice is a complex task. Most teachers have strong views on what nursing is and is not. It is not surprising then that teachers often select content on the basis of their perspective on nursing. But, as we have already seen, using one's perspective as the only basis for choice does not always ensure that the resulting content has validity for the full range of activities nurses will perform in many different contexts.

One's perspective may be narrowly confined to the specialties and may not encompass the richness and variety of nursing practice. Moreover, if too specialised, students may not see much relationship between concepts in your specialty to those in other areas of nursing.

Is it possible to express the perspective we hold so that it becomes available to others? A public and not a private perspective? A conceptualisation that can be explained through its major and minor concepts? Such a concept map is

25

advocated by Heath (1982) for curricula in nursing and by Novak (1978) for a course which an individual teacher might plan.

Having a perspective on your teaching subject (which of course arises out of your beliefs and values) is an important criterion for choosing content. Without it your teaching material will be chosen capriciously and your students will, understandably, be confused about the meaning of nursing as a subject and a service.

What is meant here is a conceptualisation of nursing which represents or captures beliefs and values about the meaning of nursing and how it should be practised. How nursing is conceptualised has been the subject of a rapidly mounting literature in recent years. There are many reasons for this. For writers such as Donaldson and Crowley, 1978, Fawcett, 1978; Stevens, 1979) the main purpose is to identify nursing as a distinctive field of knowledge. By clarifying what it is that nurses do (that if it were not done, no amount of coalescing of the service of other health professionals would replace) the unique function of nurses might be defined. The work of Virginia Henderson is so well known that you will recall immediately the familiar words of her statement on the nature of nursing (1966).

> 'The unique function of the nurse is to assist the individual, sick or well, in the performance of those activities contributing to health or recovery (or to a peaceful death) that he would perform unaided if he had the necessary strength, will or knowledge. And to do this in such a way as to help him gain independence as rapidly as possible.'

All 3 criteria may now be included in the following summary:

TABLE 2.2 : CRITERIA AND TECHNIQUES FOR DEFINING
CONTENT

Criterion	Questions	Techniques
RELEVANCE	. What does the nurse do?	Task analysis Job description
	. What is the context?	Situation analysis
	. What will the nurse do in future?	Future fore-casting
LEARNING & THE LEARNER	. What must the nurse know?	Objectives Competencies
	. How will the know-ledge be used?	Problem-solving
PERSPECTIVE OF NURSING	. What view of nursing is held	Concept mapping
	. What kind of person should the nurse be?	Conceptual framework

TECHNIQUES FOR DETERMINING CONTENT

Now that we have explained the background to
making decisions about content, we will trace each
method to show the steps involved. While the above
summary in table form might aid clarification, it
also introduces the dangers of over-simplification
and arbitrary division of the techniques into
categories. There is really a continuum of methods
rather than a separation of one technique from
another. For example, the links between task
analysis, job description, objectives and
competencies are fairly direct. Neither are tasks
carried out in a vacuum; the context or situation
also requires analysis so that the tasks or
activities are analysed against their particular
set of circumstances.

Taking the criterion of relevance first we
will use the techniques listed to answer the
questions. What does the nurse do now, in what

context, and what will be the future tasks or activities?

Activity:
Imagine that you have been asked to plan a new course in occupational health for primary health care nurses. You have decided the course should be based on the work students will do when they have completed the course. How will you proceed to define the work?

Feedback:
Depending on your experience and knowledge you could begin by finding out -
>What situations
>What functions
>What activities
>What problems
>and finally,
>What knowledge is needed to deal with
>the problems?

You may be able to supply the answers to all of these questions if you are an experienced occupational health nurse and are therefore familiar with the work conditions and environment in specific situations in occupational health. On the other hand, perhaps you are not up-to-date with this information, or you may be a community health nurse who has not actually practised in occupational health but has been shouldered with this new responsibility (because of the shortfall of trained occupational health nursing educators). Before planning your course you will need to employ one or more of the following techniques of identifying tasks and functions.

Task analysis
You may in the first instance choose to consult occupational health nurses for assistance. There are several ways of gaining information in a systematic way
>- by interviewing each one to find out the characteristics of their work - in their own words
>- by asking them to compare an already

prepared checklist of task statements with what they actually do
- by asking them to complete a daily diary sheet by recording what they did throughout each day for several days
- by inviting a group of occupational health nurses to discuss with you, in an informal meeting, their work and the purposes of their activities. In this way you will gain additional comments about the relative importance to them of the tasks they perform.

Another source of information is the observations you yourself make. There are several ways of observing tasks - from a strictly formalised method, to an open 'ethnographic' technique where the environment and tone of the situation are observed as well as the tasks. You could
- conduct a time and motion study to obtain a quantitative record of how occupational nurses spend their time
- choose a number of broad categories beforehand (e.g. interpersonal interaction, treatment, advising) then observe the particular activities carried out in each category
- became involved in occupational health work yourself, as a participant observer, collecting your impressions as well as the more objective evidence of what tasks and activities are performed in the job
- collect a number of incidents of both excellent and unsatisfactory performances which could be used as critical incidents in compiling details of what the nurse must do and know.

Another technique involves your students and becomes part of their initial project in a problem solving, or in a self-directed study course. You could
- design a project with your students to enable them to find out for themselves the elements of the work they will need to understand in order to perform later on.

29

The outcome of any of the above methods you choose will be a set of information which you can then organise into levels of activities, tasks or functions.

Taking the information gained from any of the above methods of task analysis, it would be a simple step to form a job description.

Job description

Category - Occupational Health Nurse

General situation in which the occupational health nurse will work:

The occupational health nurse is responsible for the health of workers in the plant. There is a medical officer in the district to whom referrals can be made.

Functions:

1) Conduct safety promotion programs
2) Evaluate hazards specific to industry
3) Supervise environmental monitoring
4) Assist workers to help themselves to deal with day-to-day crises.

Sample of activities within the functions:

1) Conduct safety promotion programs
   a) interview workers to assess possible allergies
   b) advise on occupational hazards specific to industry
   c) select personal protective devices
   d) fit personal safety equipment.
2) Evaluate hazards specific to industry
   a) apply knowledge of these hazards to work environment
   b) monitor occupational hazards
   c) notify hazardous levels of the work environment to authorities
   d) ... and so on.

Each one of the activities can be subdivided into more specific tasks if the level of detail you require (and your purposes in teaching the course) demands more precision in the definition of tasks. There is a great variety in the amount of detail contained in job descriptions. The rule of thumb here is simply to decide on the amount of specificity you require to assist you in deciding what to teach. (This will depend on many associated factors such as length of the course, what the students know already, what resources you have and the extent to which your colleagues in the occupational health field can assist you with on-site demonstration and field experiences.)

By now it should be fairly obvious that task analysis (narrowly employed) should not be undertaken in isolation from the constraints or the resources in the system where teaching is to take place. After all, the quantitative method of task analysis reveals what is done but not what is omitted.

Learning objectives

The importance of an analysis of tasks is that from it a set of learning objectives can be developed. Referring back to p. 27, the links between the criteria of relevance and the learner can be seen. The questions - what does the nurse do and what must the nurse learn? - lead to the formation of a learning objective, that is, those things students must know or be able to do at the completion of the course.

Activity:
In view of the controversy about the usefulness of learning objectives would you consider omitting altogether the step of constructing learning objectives now that you have a job description of the work occupational health nurses will do to assist you to choose content for your course? What implications arise from the additional step of forming a set of learning objectives?

Feedback:
This would make a fruitful topic for debate as the issues range throughout general education (Stenhouse, 1975), medical education (Simpson, 1980, Engel 1980), and nursing education (Stevens, 1979; Gibson, 1980; Quinn, 1980).

If you have made a pro and con list it might contain some of the following points:

Pro objectives	Against objectives
. directs the learner	. too limiting
. directs the teacher	. trivialises behaviour
. states the behaviour to be achieved	. describes observable behaviour only
. aids measurement	. often constructed and not used

For our purposes in this chapter, it would be difficult [as Stenhouse (1975) admits] to deny the usefulness of objectives in performance because they communicate to students, other teachers and practitioners what it is that students need to learn. This may seem a contradiction at first sight; we are trying to determine what to teach yet we are stating content in terms of what students must learn.

If we take a simple example the difference between a learning objective and a teaching objective can be illustrated.

Learning objective: On completion of instruction the student will be able to identify the hazards caused by different toxicity levels in a given environment.

Teacher objective: To ensure that students understand the hazards of different toxicity levels.

The first statement shows what the student must do and under what circumstances. Assessment to see whether the student is competent can be carried out. On the other hand the second objective relates to what the teacher will do and it is not at all clear what expectations of student performance will be required. Understandably, students and possibly the teacher will be unsure or even confused.

In summary, in order to write learning objectives, simply take each of the tasks from the job description and restate them in the form of what the student must know, be able to do, or what attitudes the student should exhibit in order to perform the task satisfactorily and show that she/he is competent.

Before leaving the topic of objectives, it is important to consider the arguments about learning objectives in nursing at present. Heath and Marson (1979) are aware of the pitfalls inherent in trying to describe the more elusive but worthwhile behaviour we require of students. Stevens (1979) points to the pressures to 'cover' content which tends to relegate content to two of the lowest levels of cognitive skills - recall and recognition. Quinn (1980) gives examples of objectives at all taxonomic levels of the cognitive, affective and psychomotor scales, while Reilly (1980) presents objectives from the perspective of the nursing process so that the stages of Assessment, Planning, Intervention and Evaluation have learning objectives which generalise across many different patient care problems.

One final but important comment is appropriate, that is that the decision to use, or not use objectives relates to the curriculum design and structure of the total course. If, for example, the course is to feature mastery learning then objectives are required to enable criterion referenced assessment of mastery to be accomplished. As has been mentioned earlier (p.31) stating clinical learning objectives enables a distinction to be made between what is required to be done (e.g. to conduct an interview) and what is required to be learnt as a result of the doing (e.g. compare your progress in interviewing using a prepared learning guide).

It may be helpful to pause at this point to review the progress we have made in answering the questions related to relevance in the Table 2. 2. Only one question - What does the nurse do? - has been addressed. But by exploring the techniques of task analysis and job description that could be used to answer that question, we found that the criterion of the learner and learning were also involved - What must the nurse know?

Situation analysis

Returning to the criterion of relevance, and the question - What is the context? - we are reminded that professional performance does not occur within a vacuum. There is no mystery here, if the client, the task and the setting are considered together. Moreover, the tasks and functions identified through observation (or any of the other methods) need to be regarded as part of the environment in which they are performed. Take the illustration of the occupational health nurse once more. It would be ludicrous to accept a list of tasks to be performed without a description of the environment because they interact with each other.

'Identifying the hazards caused by different toxicity levels' involves not only a measurement of toxicity levels and a knowledge of their harmful effects but also the awareness of anxiety levels of workers, the heating, lighting and ventilation of the plant and also whether the pattern of communication of workers and management is cooperative or confrontational.

At once the question will arise how does this assist me to decide what I am to teach? Laduca (1975) has constructed a grid called 'professional competence situation universe' where a 3-dimensional model is used to depict the client, the clinical problem and the setting. This is a helpful approach as it makes possible the integration of these three components instead of treating each one as a separate subject. A number of situations are chosen and the relevant content about the client, the problem and the setting is identified. For example taking the objective - 'identifying the hazards caused by different toxicity levels' a situation where factory workers are exposed to toxic fumes during the manufacture of rubber tyres would be identified. The situation would be described, in full, the characteristics of the workers and the setting included and the problem of hazards of toxic gas would be determined.

Competencies
The approach just described is an appropriate way to develop competencies. They represent another technique for deriving content for teaching.

Activity:
Taking the occupational health example once more, develop a competency from the information below:

Activity	Client	Situation	Problems
Identify hazards caused by different toxicity levels	All employees	Small factory; Sympathetic management	Absenteeism Fatigue. Depression

Feedback:
A competency, or the ability to perform a set of activities, or to enact a role adequately or effectively is based on an integration of content. The characteristics of the client, the description of the immediate surroundings and events, the goal to be achieved and the standard of performance to be reached are all part of the competency. That is to say that **situations** rather than subjects are the basis for deciding what to teach.

It is possible to devise a set of competencies to cover the situations a competent nurse must be prepared to manage and then select the content that must be learned and practised.

In the chosen example a suggested competency would be:
Competency:
Collect, analyse and report on data pertaining to toxicity levels and employee health and report results with recommendations to the appropriate authority.

Future forecasting

Many nurse teachers believe that it is not enough to develop content on the basis of current practice, that relevance extends to preparing the graduates of a course to have a knowledge of present and future health care and health-care trends. Deciding what to teach needs a different technique from those we have already discussed.

Activity:
Imagine you have been invited to provide a projection of what will be required by occupational health nurses in the future. The company has decided to expand its operation and to diversify its activities. The manager has said he requires nurses who will meet the challenges of the future and wants you to set up a continuing education course. How will you decide what to teach?

Feedback:
Perhaps the first thing you would do is to interview the company's management and planning departments to ascertain the time-constraints they are working in. You could also seek information on the type of diversification of activities they are planning and the goals they have set.

Armed with that information you could then select a number of experts to form a sample for a future forecasting exercise. The sample could contain occupational health nurses, community nurses, company personnel, health department and nurse education representatives.

Bevis (1973) viewed current health care trends in the light of predictions about changes in society and society's way of coping, and drew up a detailed forecast of possible changes in the future. This was then used as a basis for selection of content.

A technique known as Delphi Probe (Sullivan and Brye, 1983) can be used. The Delphi technique is a tool using sequential questionnaires. After the first round of questionnaires have been returned, the responses are analysed, coalesced and returned to the same sample for the next round of questions. Repeating this once more, the final responses reveal the crystallized opinions of the experts.

Sullivan and Brye (1983) used a Delphi technique to guide them in forecasting the future role of the nurse in the year 2000. Their findings are that nurses will become more involved in prevention, patient education, psycho-social intervention as well as technology.

An important point is made by Bevis who points

out that it is still necessary to ask - 'what are the activities or behaviours that the forecasted future changes will require in order to select specific content and experiences'.

An outline of the Delphi probe technique used to select content is given below:

Ask experts about projected changes
Recycle answers to the same experts
Repeat twice
Compile the end results into future forecasts
Identify tasks, activities, functions, behaviours
Select content.

Problem-solving

How will the student use the knowledge that she/he must know? Referring back to Table 2.2 we nominated problem-solving as an appropriate technique. (Actually, in attempting a full answer to the question, we are in deep water and the issues raised by such a question are treated in Chapter 3.) So, in this chapter, we are looking at problem-solving as a way of determining what to teach.

Activity:
You are planning to use the problem-solving method in teaching your students. What advantages do you see in using this method in your course?

Feedback:
If you are teaching in a problem-based course, naturally your students will use a problem-based method of learning. [For a detailed discussion see Barrows & Tamblyn (1980). Written by a physician and a nurse, the text deals with the development and implementation of the method.]

On the other hand you might consider the advantages of a problem-solving method are attractive if your students use nursing process as a method of nursing practice. Your view here would be that the two complement each other.

Disadvantages you might also have noted are inherent in a problem-solving method that has become 'de-problemised'. Geach (1974) pointed out what she believed to be an intellectualising of problem-solving. Students were taught a method which had little reflection in day-to-day dealing with real problems. Her view in 'The problem-solving technique: is it relevant to nursing practice?' was aimed at bringing teachers and clinicians together to resolve the dilemma.

Another disadvantage you might have come across is the weakening of the students' opportunity to learn through problem-solving by prescribing beforehand what pathway should be followed. This is a considerable curtailment of initiative (and is antithetical to problem-solving) if it is applied in the form of a checklist to every patient.

Yet another disadvantage to learning to nurse occurs when the problem-solving method is used to rehearse the student's responses before there is an opportunity for applying problem-solving in the real situation.

Allen (1977) shows two ways of teaching in the problem-solving mode:
1) Students can be prepared beforehand to meet several situations
2) the teacher can provide the means by which the student and patient can interact together in a problem-solving way.

An example of the first method is where teacher and student rehearse what will be said to the patient, possible replies by the patient, and how the patient will be prepared. Allen comments that 'training a nurse to respond to artificial situations of this nature is in conflict with the problem-solving approach' (p.28). The alternative suggested by Allen is the second method where nurses learn to nurse patients whose problems are less well known and understood (See Allen for detailed account of the two types of teaching).

The topic of clinical decision-making is exercising the research skills of nurses (Anderson, 1976; Bennett,1976) and it is likely that when more results are produced to enlighten teachers about the way nurses make decisions, the teaching of problem identification and resolution will change.

Returning to the original intent of this section - determining content using the problem-solving method - and using problem-solving as in (2) above, it is apparent that the student and the patient, not the teacher, determine the content.

The content is not prescribed beforehand but is identified by the student who realises what information she/he requires after interviewing, or discussing how the patient views the problem. In determining content, the student learns to distinguish important from lesser important material and also where or from whom the information may be obtained. In effect the student learns what knowledge and skills are required and how she/he will use that knowledge and skill.

Not all problem-solving can be taught on-site with the patient or client.

Activity:
In the classroom, what content would you be able to supply?

Feedback:
Again, the student will determine most of the content in a true problem-solving method. The teacher provides the resources.

For example, a computer assisted program could be used where the student gives alternative responses to meet the problem.

Another set of resources can be supplied in the form of a patient study where a patients' initial history and record is supplied. The student then determines what additional information is required.

A third method is an 'in-basket' set of materials where the material relevant to a problem is supplied. The student must identify the problem(s), give a rationale and a set of actions to be used in the resolution. Examples of resource materials are community situations such as:
- the local council's ruling in respect of housing
- a disdavantaged resident's letter to the daily paper
- a domiciliary nurse's report on a terminally ill patient in the housing affected
- a letter to the local hospital from the patient's family asking for increased resources
- ... and so on

39

For the teacher, the selection of content becomes the selection of resources.

Concept mapping

What view of nursing is held? What kind of person should the nurse be? These questions are related to the criterion we named 'having a perspective on nursing' in order to determine content for teaching.

A concept map is a way of representing the central ideas within a field of knowledge or a discipline of study. By drawing a map which links the concepts (or main ideas, or points of interest) the relationship among the concepts can be linked and described. It is the linking of the concepts which is of great interest to nurses at present. As we shall see later in this section stating the relationship between two concepts is a way of forming a principle.

In nurse education a framework made up of concepts and principles (or a conceptual framework) serves two important purposes. First, as a basis for curriculum development, and for the selection of content, teaching methods and modes of practice. Second, as a basis for the development of nursing theory. When the principles (or propositions) are tested the conceptual framework then becomes a theoretical framework and from it begins the development of a theory.

For our purposes in this text we are interested in concept mapping as a stimulus for generating content for a course, and on a smaller scale for a lesson. Additionally, by using the method of concept mapping students are able themselves to identify the relationships between concepts and to begin to generate principles which they will later test for their application to practice. Concept mapping is, therefore, not only a way of determining content but a method of learning to transfer knowledge into practice.

Why not try constructing a concept map step by step in order to trace the features and process of developing a map?

Activity:
Below is a selected reading from a text on nursing theory. Identify the relevant concepts

by underlining them or by writing them on small cards.

'REALISM VERSUS CONCEPTUALISM

Very generally, two opposing kinds of "theory" are evident in the literature on nursing theory: realism and conceptualism. It is important that the reader of theory recognize and differentiate these two views, for they are different and irreconcilable. In realism, one believes that the world exists "out there" independent of the knower. Research and theory seek to discover the nature of that reality. In conceptualism, "reality" does not exist independent of the knower. Invention, rather than discovery, is dominant in conceptualism, whereas understanding, rather than construction, typifies realism. These two differing views of theory impact upon the methods and tools employed in research. This is why it is crucial to distinguish between them.

Until recently, nursing has compartmentalized "reality" by creating departments of medical-surgical, obstetrical, pediatric, psychiatric, and public health nursing. At present, however, different concepts are calling for new perceptions of the nursing world - perceptions that see a different world to be acted on and call for a different constellation of nursing acts. Distributive or episodic nursing, nursing based on a health-illness continuum, or nursing based on life phase, for example, cuts across categories previously seen as describing the nursing world. These instantiations of nursing exemplify conceptualism, which provides different "worlds" for different eyes; each person "sees" different aspects of a complex world, dependent on some given principle of selection.'
(Stevens, 1979 p. 193-194.)

Feedback:
Your list may contain some or all of the following concepts:
    nursing theory   construction

realism   comparmentalised
conceptualism   new perceptions
existence   different constellations
knowledge   health-illness
research   life-phase
discovery   different 'worlds'
invention   different aspects
understanding

Activity:
Having made the selection of concepts the next
step is to order or rank them from the most
inclusive (general) to the least inclusive
(specific).

Feedback:
    The least inclusive concepts are often
examples given to clarify a point. In the reading
above, the examples of health-illness continuum and
life phase, medical surgical and so on, are least
inclusive concepts in the passage. Nursing theory,
the main root of the passage is the most inclusive.
Those concepts lying between are intermediate
concepts and can be assigned arbitrarily on the
map.
    Your marking of the concepts from most to
least inclusive might have taken the following
order:

Most inclusive   nursing theory literature,
                      realism, conceptualism,
                      existence   independent of answer
                      research   invention   discovery
                      construction   understanding
     different constellation
                      compartmentalised new perceptions
                      different world   medical
                      surgical   paediatric
                      psychiatric   public health
                      obstetrical   health-illness
                      continuum
Least inclusive   life phase.

Activity:
The map can now be constructed. Arrange   the

concepts with the most inclusive at the top, followed by the next most inclusive, until all the concepts have been arranged. Then establish the links between the concepts by drawing a line and stating what the relationship is between any two concepts.

Feedback:
The map does not have to be symmetrical and there is of course no right or wrong way to draw the map as inclusiveness of concepts often depends upon individual interpretation. After all, the purpose of constructing a concept map from a reading is to identify the subject matter more clearly for your own purpose.
One way in which the concepts could be linked is

FIGURE 2.1: EXAMPLE OF A CONCEPT MAP

Nursing theory
Literature

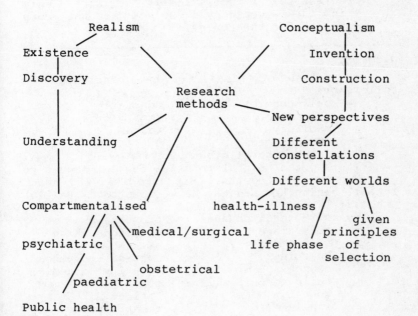

Although the reading was comparatively short the implications of the exercise for identifying what to teach from an assigned text are obvious. Again, students can also derive benefit in knowledge and skill from an analysis of written material they are required to learn.

Almost the same technique is used for constructing a concept map for a course. This time there is no assigned passage of reading. Instead, you, as a teacher preparing to teach a course, want to work on a conceptualisation of your field; a new perception and a 'different constellation of nursing acts.'

Activity:
Imagine you are planning a new set of teaching/learning sessions on rehabilitation and you want your students to realise the continuous nature of rehabilitation, its multidisciplinary character and the extension of its principle throughout the patients' progress to the home, family and work. What main ideas would you select as the core concepts for the course?

Feedback:
Your list of ideas may have included the following:

self-concept	adaptation
prevention	family/friends
mobility	values
independence	quality of life
interpersonal growth.	

It is often helpful to ask a few colleagues to do the same, or together 'brainstorm' ideas about rehabilitation and add any new concepts to the list such as:

structural changes	prosthesis
body image	decision-making
facing reality	self-help
learning	cost-effectiveness
change	security(economic)
building on positives	coping with limi-
honesty	tations
wheelchair	rehabilitation aids

When you have exhausted the ideas, identify the most and least inclusive concepts as was done in the previous exercise. Proceeding with concept mapping, link the concepts in hierarchy and state any relationships you recognise.

One way of linking the concepts would be:

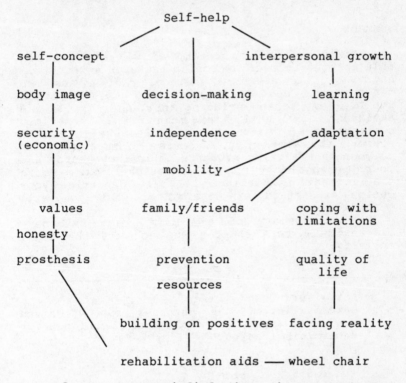

If you are satisfied that the concept map represents your major concept and the required flow of ideas you could then identify the content and practice you wish to teach.

Rehabilitation is an interesting area for concept mapping as the role of the nurse is often unclear and because of this the teaching of rehabilitation is often limited to the regime of the other health professionals. Clearly, there is a role for nursing in rehabilitation. But identifying content by conventional means, for example, psychology, sociology, orthopaedics or gerontology fails to highlight concepts of learning, decision-making, quality of life - all arising from the needs of the person and the situation rather than the professional or the academic discipline.

SUMMARY

Deciding what to teach, as we have seen in this chapter, can be a complex task for a teacher. Any one of a number of methods can be used to determine the content of your teaching. Content in the broadest sense including knowledge, skills and attitudes is what is meant and sometimes combination of several methods will assist you to achieve the aims of your course. Your particular purpose in assisting students to learn to nurse and your personal style as a teacher and as a practitioner of nursing will also determine your choice of method of determining what you will teach.

As a summary of the main points we have discussed in this chapter why not try the final activity:

Activity:
Make a list of the purposes for which you would use each of the following techniques for determining content.

Task analysis
Job description
Situation analysis
Future forecasting
Objectives
Competencies
Problem solving
Concept mapping

Feedback:
It is possible that your list will be different from the list any of your colleagues may produce in answer to the same activity. There

are no right or wrong answers. However, inappropriate use of some techniques could result in a selection of content for your course which fails to satisfy you or your students. Again your knowledge of the level and progress of your students and your appreciation of the aims of the total course will influence your choice of method. The following, therefore, is meant only as a guide.

Use task analysis if you aim to
- base your teaching on specific components of nursing practice e.g. demonstrations
- develop specific behavioural objectives for your students
- identify the knowledge, skills and attitudes in a particular activity
- identify components of the nurse's role in total patient care.

Use situational analysis if you aim to
- include the context and the environment of nursing activities in your course
- emphasise to students the importance of the patient's background (e.g. family and work) in the planning for and giving of care
- base your selection of content on the problems of patients rather than a series of separated subjects.

Use job description if you aim to
- determine the specific steps in a task or activity
- provide the student with the elements of the work they will be required to do
- direct your teaching towards the tasks and activities expected of your students.

Use future forecasting if you aim to
- plan a course to meet the future as well as the immediate needs of students.
- prepare students for change
- stimulate your teaching by keeping up-to-date with trends in your field

Use objectives if you aim to
- specify a number of levels of achievement expected of students

47

- provide a learning guide to students
- define the limits of the course
- provide criteria for assessment.

Use competencies if you aim to
- include qualitative as well as quantitative dimensions of care
- provide a basis for interdisciplinary content
- include sets of activities to be achieved rather than specific tasks
- provide for integration of tasks and clinical situations.

Use problem-solving if you aim to
- complement the general aims of a problem-based course
- prepare students for problem-based nursing practice
- involve students in determining what they need to know in resolving problems.

Use concept mapping if you aim to
- identify a set of concepts to represent a patient problem
- cut across subject boundaries
- integrate knowledge from several fields
- present nursing knowledge so that it transfers to practice.

Chapter 3.

HELPING STUDENTS LEARN

The purpose of this chapter is to examine some aspects of learning theory which are relevant to the education of nurses.

When you have finished this chapter you should be able to use relevant aspects of learning theories as the basis for decisions about the way you arrange your teaching to help students learn.

There are many excellent books which deal with specific theories of learning or which integrate or provide overviews of the major theories. It is not possible within a single chapter to deal with the details and the interrelationships of those theories. The purpose of this chapter is therefore to sketch an outline of current beliefs about how students learn and to provide a framework for decisions teachers make. References will be provided throughout and are recommended if you wish to follow up any aspects more thoroughly.

Aspects of specific teaching methods which are frequently used in nurse education are discussed in the following chapter, and it is true that most teachers operate within a context of traditional teaching methods such as lectures, practical classes of some sort or another, and small group work. However, even within those traditional methods there is room for innovation and application of ideas intended to maximise the learning students experience. The first step toward such innovations is for teachers to ask themselves 'How do students learn?' and to base their teaching on their answers to that question. You do not have to be an expert in educational theory to answer that question. All teachers have also been students for considerable periods of time and have experienced both effective and ineffective learning episodes. So the answer to the question 'How do students learn?' begins with your own experiences.

Activity:
Think about your learning career as a nursing student and as a graduate.
Can you remember a learning experience which was particularly effective?
What made it effective, write down as many things about it as you can remember.
Sometimes it is easier to recall learning experiences which did not work well, is there some topic which you always found difficult?
How were you taught about that topic, what factors inhibited your learning? Write down the reasons why you feel you were unable to learn effectively.

Feedback:
Obviously there can be no 'model feedback' for this activity because learning is a personal experience and not all learners will require the same conditions for learning. In fact that is one of the most important things for teachers to remember - **there are differences among students which affect their learning.**
The factors you have listed might include factors within yourself which influenced your ability or readiness to learn, factors within the environment or context, or factors within the subject matter itself which helped or hindered your learning. It is artificial to separate conditions for learning into discrete categories since there is considerable interaction between personal, contextual and topic characteristics, however for ease of presentation those categories will be used as the basic organising structure for the remainder of this chapter. It will become clear as we proceed that there is considerable overlap among the factors discussed, and some concepts such as motivation and feedback for example, feature in all categories.

CONDITIONS FOR LEARNING — WITHIN THE STUDENT

Activity:
Drawing on your experience as a learner and a teacher identify the major factors within the individual which influence learning.

Feedback:
Factors within the student which may influence learning are numerous. Your list may include the following factors:

Motivation to learn
Interest in the topic
General ability or intelligence
Aptitude for the topic or specific skills
Learning style or preferred learning strategies.

You may also have listed other factors, or used different terms than the ones used here. There is some overlap among the abstract concepts which have been developed to define individual differences among learners. For example the unitary concept of intelligence as measured by intelligence testing reflects motivation, general abilities, specific skills, cognitive strategies and cultural differences. Similarly 'personality tests' measure aspects of abilities, motivation, strategies, preferences and cultural characteristics. The important thing to remember about such definitions of individual differences is that, while they are concepts which may be useful in planning learning experiences which accommodate to individual needs, they are usually not sufficiently precise or reliable to be used as predictors of student performance. Allocation of tertiary level students to 'ability groups' may be convenient for the teacher but the benefits for the students are debatable. While prescription of specific remedial activities may enhance certain aspects of the students' performance, other aspects of ability grouping reinforce teachers' lowered expectations of lower level groups and poor self-concepts of students in those groups, resulting in a 'self-fulfilling prophecy' which may actually impede the progress of those students.

Individual differences contribute to students' opportunities to learn from each other and they present a challenge to teachers who are interested in getting to know their students and in helping each student to maximise his or her learning potential. The nature of individual differences is extremely complex and attempts to develop general rules to assist teachers to link specific teaching strategies with specific individual abilities have met with limited success despite considerable research efforts (for a review of research into aptitude-treatment interactions see Cronbach & Snow, 1977). Nevertheless, teachers will be assisted by a general awareness of the nature of individual differences and their potential influence on learning.

Motivation

Motivation can be defined in many ways but for our purposes we will take it to mean the desire or wish to learn. The desire to learn can be generated by many factors, some of which are more relevant for some students and some learning contexts than others.

Activity:
What motivates your students to learn what you teach them?
What motivates you to continue your professional learning?
Do your reasons for wanting to learn differ from those of your students in any significant ways? What makes the difference if there is one?

Feedback:
The list of factors which motivate individuals to learn is endless and very dependent on specific circumstances, however one important distinction can be made which provides a framework for understanding the nature of motivation. That is the distinction between a desire to learn which is generated from within the individual and a desire

to learn which is generated by external influences.

Traditional educational programs provide quite a high degree of **external motivation** in the form of barrier examinations, grades, rules for admission to, and exclusion from courses, and expressions of praise or criticism from teachers. By contrast **internal motivation** arises in situations where the learner has an intrinsic interest in the learning task, pursuing personal educational goals to increase a sense of personal mastery and professional competence. While the two types of motivation are certainly not mutually exclusive teachers frequently observe that students 'are only interested in what they will be asked in the exams'. New students begin with a degree of internal motivation to learn to be competent nurses, but the facts of survival teach them that such goals are a subsequent issue to passing examinations and pleasing the teachers, and external motivation gradually takes precedence for most students. Once the students have graduated and become practising professionals however, most of the external imperative to learn is removed and graduates must rediscover their sources of internal motivation in order to maintain professional competence. Some do so quite successfully but some have been so disenchanted with learning to pass the examinations that they have little desire to continue their learning and seek only enough professional education to keep them safe. In the above activity you may have noticed that your reasons for learning are related to your personal needs and responsibilities, while to some extent at least your students' reasons for learning are related to the requirement to satisfy external conditions before personal needs or interests. The task for teachers is to create conditions for learning in which students' internal motivation is recognised and encouraged to develop, and in which sources of external motivation are kept in proper perspective.

Maslow (1943) has proposed a theory of motivation which is a useful conceptual framework. He has suggested a hierarchy of five basic needs beginning with the need for physiological satisfaction and progressing through the need for safety, love, self-esteem and self-actualisation. Comparison of sources of motivation in nursing education with this hierarchy reveals that the external motivation described above relates mainly to the need for safety and to some extent the need for 'love' or approval from one's teachers and colleagues. Internal motivation as described above relates more closely to the need for self-esteem which leads to a feeling of self-confidence, worth and capability; and to the need for self-actualisation, the process by which one comes to depend on the self rather than to identify with others and to rely, when necessary, on personal standards independently of external demands, (Lovell, p. 111, 1980). Given this definition self-actualisation is clearly to be encouraged in the education of nurses.

Interest in the topic
       Interest in the topic to be learned is related to motivation and the desire to learn. It is inevitable that levels of interest will vary among students who will be influenced by a multitude of factors such as personal preferences and abilities, like or dislike of the teacher, the presence of competing events such as examinations in another subject, or even the time of day or season. You may have little control over some of these factors which impinge on the students' interest, however a major factor which you can do something about is the perceived relevance of what the students have to learn. Pressured by competing demands on their time students have to make decisions about learning priorities - one criterion they use to help them decide is **relevance.** Students judge the relevance of a topic according to how well they can perceive a relationship between that topic and their ultimate goal of becoming a nurse. Consequently ward work is seen to be very relevant and generates a lot of interest. Basic science courses when taught in isolation from clinical practice or examples have a more tenuous relationship to the ultimate goal and are perceived as less relevant hurdles to be surmounted rather than integral parts of nursing education. Teachers can increase the perceived relevance of topics at any stage of training by attention to the **sequence** in which subject matter is presented. For example traditional structures of disciplines tend to progress from basic facts to combinations of those

facts into general principles and then application of those principles in solution of problems. Not surprisingly, teachers often follow this same sequence in their teaching because it is logical and familiar, unfortunately it may be less motivating and interesting for the students who cannot grasp the relevance of the basic facts and principles until they have experienced the problems to which those facts and principles will be applied. Problem-based learning experiences (see Chapter 6), correlation classes, vertical integration of subjects and conceptual frameworks such as the nursing process (Yura & Walsh, 1978) are all attempts to use alternative approaches to the sequence of instruction which demonstrate relevance and promote interest. At a more basic level asking students questions or giving them problems to solve stimulates curiosity and generates more interest than does merely providing information as a collection of facts.

General ability or intelligence

While general ability or intelligence in its general sense undoubtedly influences the capacity of individuals to learn, the specific effects are impossible to determine simply because we have no adequate definitions or criteria for such general abilities (Lovell, p. 99, 1980). Individuals differ in their innate potential for learning along innumerable dimensions, but research into the intellectual development of children constantly reminds us of the enormous influence of environmental factors on the realisation of that potential (Blank & Solomon, 1969). Some educators believe that, given appropriate learning experiences 'all or almost all students can master what they are taught' (Block, p.3. 1971). This should certainly be true in nursing education where a selection process has been used to decide which students will be accepted for training. In professional training courses where academic performance is invariably one criterion used for selection, teachers have little grounds for attributing poor student performance to 'lack of ability'.

Aptitudes and specific skills

Aptitudes and specific skills are components

55

of general ability which are able to be identified and defined. To a certain extent they may be innate but they are also certainly shaped by training and experience. For example innate musical talent may differentiate the concert pianist from the mediocre player, but no amount of innate talent will create a concert pianist from someone who begins musical training late in life. Some nursing schools have attempted to identify specific aptitudes and skills which are believed essential in the profession of nursing and to incorporate those into selection procedures. Ability to communicate effectively is one such aptitude, another is arithmetical calculation. On the other hand, some aptitudes are expected to develop in training and become part of the learning objectives rather than criteria for selection.

Activity:
Which aptitudes or specific skills do you expect students to exhibit or develop in the area that you teach? What difficulties do students encounter in achieving those objectives? Do some achieve the desirable level of skill faster than others?

Feedback:
The last question in that activity is a leading question, since one conception of aptitude defines it as the characteristic which predicts the rate at which a student can learn a given task rather than the level of learning possible. Out of this idea developed the concept of mastery learning which proposes that, discounting 5% of individuals with specific disabilities for certain subjects, 95% of students can learn a subject to a high level of mastery if given sufficient learning time and appropriate types of help. Some students will require more effort, time and help to achieve the criterion level or the level of minimum competence required. The teacher's task is to find ways of reducing the learning time for slower students so that it does not become prohibitively slow, and to offer enrichment experiences for those students who proceed at a faster pace (Bloom, 1971).

Mastery learning is a very important concept in nursing education where professional responsibilities demand that all registered nurses have achieved <u>at least</u> a minimum level of competence in central aspects of their role. Core curricula define those competences which students <u>must</u> master and the level of satisfactory performance. Once those objectives have been achieved students can progress to develop skills and knowledge in 'should know' areas then 'nice to know' areas (Abbatt, 1980).

Aptitudes for learning in specific areas are not static and may progress with the development of the individual, maintaining and strengthening necessary aptitudes is therefore a factor which teachers should consider in deciding how to help students learn. Flexibility needs to be built into learning experiences to allow for differential rates of progress and different levels of need for information or practice. One approach to providing this flexibility is the use of self-paced modules or learning units which allow students to progress through subject matter at their own speed and to use their contact with the teacher for higher level learning such as comprehension and problem solving rather than simply the acquisition of basic information or skills (Cyrs, 1976; Kochman, 1976; WHO, 1976).

A related factor which teachers should bear in mind is the 'readiness' of students to undertake learning in certain areas. **Readiness** may relate to aptitudes, previous experience, interest or personal development and it is to be expected that various levels of readiness will exist among students and that learning experiences may have to take account of that variation. For example, not all students may be ready to take part in a discussion about care of the dying patient so the discussion should be structured in a way which allows an atmosphere of comfort and trust and which introduces the topic at a level which is meaningful to all participants. Some students may be ready to deal with factual issues before emotional issues, some students may need to deal with emotional issues before they can address the technical or factual issues. Experienced teachers, like experienced nurses can call on their professional judgement to help them analyse the situation and formulate a management plan, on the spot if necessary.

There are no hard and fast rules to help teachers adapt teaching to students' individual needs since too many variables intervene to allow accurate prescription of strategies. However, if you are aware of, and sensitive to, the variations in readiness and aptitudes which occur even within an academically homogeneous group you will maintain sufficient flexibility to help all your students learn and achieve the required level of competence.

Learning style and strategies

Learning style (sometimes called cognitive style) is a newer concept of individual differences which is relevant to education. Cognitive style is basically the ways in which people process information. It incorporates such things as the ways in which sensory stimuli are perceived and interpreted, the strategy which the individual uses in forming concepts, and solving problems, and the approaches an individual takes to learning a given body of material. For example, some people tend to gather information systematically and arrive at solutions to problems by logical deduction (focusing), other people tend to begin with a few educated guesses and gather information as they proceed (scanning) (Bruner, Goodnow & Austin, 1956); some seek a single right or best answer to questions or problems (convergers), some prefer to cast the net widely seeking potential solutions in innovative areas (divergers). Hudson (1968) has described 'syllabus bound' learners who happily accept restrictions of a formal syllabus and aim for good examination results, and 'syllabus free' learners who have intellectual interests extending beyond the set syllabus. Witkin, Lewis, Hertzman, Machover, Meissener & Wagner (1954) described field dependence as the tendency to rely on external cues for determining the position of the body in space, and field independence as the tendency to rely on internal proprioceptive cues. Field dependence and independence have subsequently been correlated with styles of visual perception, intellectual function, personality and career preferences; a comprehensive review of the educational implications of this cognitive style is provided by Witkin, Moore, Goodenough & Cox (1977). Pask (1976) has categorised learning strategies as serialist - in which the learner prefers to build up a total picture by accumulating and assembling details, and holist - in which the learner prefers to gain an overview of the topic as a general structure in which the details fall into place. Kagan (1965) has observed that some learners, when confronted with a problem delay before offering a solution which is usually correct - they take the time to internally evaluate potential solutions - Kagan called this reflectivity. In contrast some learners offer solutions rapidly which are often wrong, relying on the teacher or some other external source to evaluate their efforts - this tendency was designated as impulsivity. A good review of the individual differences in cognitive styles is available in Messick (1976).

A critical study of the details of these dimensions of cognitive styles may lead to the suspicion that many researchers are using different terms to describe very similar tendencies which overlap considerably with older notions such as creativity, intelligence and personality variables, nevertheless the dimensions do offer some insights into the complexities involved in perceiving, processing and retaining information in a form in which it is able to be effectively used. Without a doubt learners are very active in the process of learning.

Learning 'is an active process of mind on experience' (Wilson, p. 25, 1981). By contrast many traditional teaching strategies such as lectures and tests of factual recall are based on a passive model of learning in which 'knowledge as a copy of reality .... has to be committed in its present form to the memory of the learner' (Wilson, p. 24). Piaget (1971) has described learning as essentially a simultaneous process of assimilation and accommodation in which the learner incorporates the learned object or event while also taking account of its peculiarities and adapting existing cognitive structures to achieve a good fit. Ausubel (1960) has extended this idea with the suggestion that learning can be improved by the provision of 'advance organisers' which help the student to activate relevant parts of his or her cognitive structures in readiness for the assimilation and accommodation which forms the crucial part of the learning task.

The following activity will provide an example of what is meant by **advance organisers.**

Activity:
Read this list of syllables and then close your eyes and try to recall as many as you can: MAI, CON, DEL, MAR, MAS, PEN, RHO, VER, GEO, FLO, VIR.

Feedback:
Probably you tried to make some sense out of the syllables as an aid to memory. Given the task of learning nonsense syllables people usually try to link them to words or link them together into meaningful sentences or work out some type of code to fit into their memory (or cognitive structure). In fact these syllables are the first three letters of the names of eleven states on the east coast of the USA. If you had known that at the beginning would you have found it easier to learn the list? Probably your answer is 'yes'. If you had been given that advance organiser you would have been able to call up the relevant parts of your existing knowledge and fit the new learning into it in a way which would have facilitated your ability to recall the syllables. The advance organiser would have transformed the syllables from meaningless to meaningful information.

What does this mean for the teacher? It means that learning will only occur if the subject or skill or attitude to be learned has meaning for the student and can be fitted into what the student already knows from education or experience. Learning which cannot be locked into existing knowledge or cognitive structure is short-lived and may not be retained in useable form. Once again however individual differences among students will create problems for the teacher who cannot be expected to know which learning styles are preferred by which students, nor which aspects of the learning are likely to be meaningful and which will require special activities to ensure that they become useable parts of the students' accumulated experience.

Activity:
Make a list of the strategies you could use in your teaching to help students process and incorporate information or skills in a form which has meaning for them and which will be retained for future application.

Feedback:
There are probably many more ways to achieve **meaningful learning** than the ones listed below, however these should be feasible in most teaching contexts:

1. Provide a **pretest** of knowledge, skills or attitudes to give both you and the students an idea of their existing position in relation to the learning to be undertaken.

2. Suggest **reading assignments** before class so that all students have at least thought about the issues to be discussed and perhaps related them to things they already know or problems they have already encountered.

3. Introduce topics at a level which you can be sure is understood by everybody, use **familiar examples** to introduce unfamiliar concepts e.g. the analogy between the heart and a mechanical pump, or the knee joint and a hinge.

4. **Use materials, case histories,** discussion topics, role plays etc. to which students can relate on a personal basis. Most students have some experience with illness among their own families and friends and can draw on these experiences to approach clinical problems even at a very early stage in their training.

5. Provide **alternative learning methods** such as self-instructional materials, or handouts instead of, or in addition to, traditional methods. The provision of alternative resources and methods which suit different

learning styles and preferences helps to improve student performance (Lesser, 1972).

6. Ensure that group activities have sufficient **built-in flexibility** to accommodate to the needs of the individuals in the group as well as sufficient structure to encourage task completion.

7. **Consult with students** in the setting of objectives for their learning. This option is perhaps more feasible in areas of the course which are not considered to be core, for example elective terms, practicum experiences, or group assignments. This type of approach in which the learning objectives and criteria for satisfactory performance are determined jointly by teachers and students is called **contracting** (Knowles, 1975). Contracting provides valuable opportunities for the development of personal strategies for structuring learning, and the capacity for self-evaluation.

8. Encourage an **enquiring approach to the process** as well as the content of learning. Discussion of the processes by which students arrived at an answer to a question, or a solution to a problem, or a plan for management makes learning strategies explicit and gives students a chance to compare their personal strategies with their teachers' and colleagues' strategies, and where appropriate, to develop more efficient and effective approaches.

9. Actively **discourage rote memorisation** of facts and lists by setting examinations which test understanding and the ability to apply knowledge.

10. Plan your teaching to include as much **active participation** by students as possible. Only by working on, and with new knowledge will they be able to make it their own knowledge.

CONDITIONS IN THE LEARNING CONTEXT

Activity:
Drawing on your experience as a learner and
teacher identify the major factors within the
learning context or environment which
influence learning.

Feedback:
The **learning context** can be defined as those
factors which affect the attitudes of your students
to each other, to you, your subject and to learning
itself. They are difficult factors to define and
their exact nature will differ very much from
culture to culture, but they can be broadly divided
into physical aspects of the environment and
psychological or emotional aspects of the
environment.

Do your students enjoy learning? Are they
interested to learn and motivated to study because
of that interest rather than the threat of
examinations? Do they cooperate with each other? Do
they feel free to approach you for help and to
discuss their learning deficiencies with you? Do
they feel safe to discuss emotional matters and
attitudes with their fellow students? Are they
receiving the individual attention that some may
need more than others? Are you aware of some of
their individual needs and how to help them?

Attitudes to education have changed over the
past few years, under the influence of philosophies
held by people like Maslow (1943), Rogers (1969)
and Bruner (1962) who stressed the personal
development aspects of education and who advocated
that conditions should be created which allow
students sufficient 'freedom to learn' unhindered
by rigid conceptions of the learning task as an
information transfer exercise. Dewey (1917) had
expressed similar ideas much earlier and more
recent and radical approaches have been taken by
Illich (1971) and Freire (1970). All are based on
the philosophy that people have a natural desire to
learn and will undertake learning in the pursuit of
personal competence, self-esteem, self-actualisation and enjoyment. Knowles (1975) has applied

the same principles to the study of adult learning in particular and has concluded that adults are motivated to learn in order to solve problems which have personal relevance for them. All of these educators have criticised aspects of traditional education which stress external rewards for learning and which leave little room for creativity and personal development alongside the achievement of set learning objectives.

More traditional views of learning held that students were in nursing school to learn, not to enjoy themselves or to express their individuality. In contrast, modern theories about learning suggest that an investment in the emotional well-being of students will pay off in the form of more positive attitudes towards learning, and ultimately towards nursing responsibilities. Planning for appropriate learning conditions cannot bring about learning if students are not motivated to learn or not courageous enough to seek help with their problems. Admittedly this approach comes more naturally to some teachers than others and many good teachers have always been aware of the importance of the learning context and have developed personal ways of creating it. Orton (1983) carried out research into learning climate in wards and concluded that 'good learning environments can be identified as those displaying teamwork, good communication and a concern for individual students and their learning needs.'

Activity:
You will have developed some ways of creating a comfortable and productive learning context in your classroom - in other words, you will be aware of certain actions that you take which help both you and your students to work with the subject matter in a way that makes learning effective.

Write down some of the methods that you use. Include physical factors as well as social or psychological ones.

Feedback:

<u>Physical factors</u>
     Under physical factors you may have listed the following:

1.   Adequate lighting, ventilation, seating and temperature control.

2.   Seating arrangements - flexibility in seating arrangements allows for the creation of environments to suit specific learning contexts, for example students seated in a circle find it easier and more comfortable to have a discussion. If you wish to join the discussion you should join the circle. Seating arrangements which place you at the front of the class ensure that you do all of the talking. Of course that might be desirable for some contexts but probably not for all.

3.   Learning materials and resources - these increase the flexibility of classroom activity and allow a variety of approaches to learning with the teacher playing a greater or lesser role as is appropriate (see Chapter 6).

4.   Sufficient learning spaces to allow students to pursue private study or group activities in relative comfort and close proximity to any necessary resources.

5.   Convenient and frequent access to hospitals or other institutions in which practical training is occurring. Easy access and allocation of a student common room increases students' feeling of belonging in the institution and contributing to its function.

<u>Social factors</u>
     Under social or psychological factors you may have listed the following:

1.   Your own personality - Most of us have to operate with the personality we have because it is difficult and may not be desirable to change. However, any teacher should be able to create warmth in interaction with a class -

this can be done, for example, by avoiding insulting or sarcastic remarks. Walking among students in class or sitting with them will decrease your distance from them and give the impression of approachability.

2. Maintaining a working atmosphere in the class is important but there is room for some relaxation to allow for questions, discussion and minor diversions from the topic to explore an unexpected outcome of the lesson. If this type of behaviour is accepted by students and teachers then students are encouraged to think more about the topic and to gain confidence in their own abilities.

3. Treating students as individuals may be difficult with a large class but it should be attempted whenever possible. Learning students' names, taking time to praise work well done or to assist with work poorly done will increase the students' motivation to work well and will also provide them with a model to follow when they are teachers themselves.

4. Avoiding harsh criticism helps to create trust and students feel more prepared to risk making comments which they want to try out with the teacher and class. It is true that this is sometimes difficult, teachers are only human and students sometimes disappoint them badly. However, while students certainly need to be told when they are wrong or when they are behaving in an undesirable manner, such criticism should be constructive rather than destructive. Point out what they have done wrong and how they should do it correctly, but try to avoid personal insults such as accusations of stupidity.

5. Encouraging students to develop internal standards by which to judge their own efforts increases their level of internal motivation and personal and professional development. Ask for their opinion of their work before you offer yours. Discuss their goals with them and offer constructive feedback on their appropriateness.

6. Setting goals with students which are cooperative or individualistic rather than competitive. Johnson & Johnson (1974) have described these three goal structures in education. The competitive goal structure which predominates in traditional educational practice evaluates students against the performance of their fellows. Professional nurses, as we have already seen, need to be able to develop internal goals and standards and to achieve mastery in specific responsibilities - this requires individualistic goal structures in which students are assessed against their achievement of personal goals determined on the basis of individual needs. On the other hand, nurses will work as part of a health care team and should be familiar with working within cooperative goal structures where individuals are assessed on the basis of their contribution to the tasks of their group.

7. Being aware of the process of professional socialisation. Simpson (1979) has defined the dimensions of socialisation as cognitive preparation to perform the role, orientations to the demands of the role and the appropriate behaviour to meet those demands, and motivation to make the transition from training to work. Opportunities to work alongside practising nurses and acceptance by them as junior colleagues are important to the development of the students' concepts of themselves as nurses. Care should be taken to ensure that the practices and principles taught in the school or classroom are relevant to the realities of practice and either reinforce professional values displayed in practice or explicitly prepare students for divergent value orientations that they might encounter in different environments. Simpson, in a sociological study of one nursing college in the United States concluded that entering students endorsed views that fitted well with the conception of the ideal nurse that the school wanted to prepare but that the process of their education shifted their views towards a bureaucratic conception of nursing, ideally

67

opposed by the faculty. The curriculum and student assignments on wards emphasised technical, task-oriented nursing and students developed orientations consistent with this emphasis. The implication is that students conform to the real demands made upon them rather than to abstract ideals presented or rehearsed in theoretical contexts.

This list is by no means complete, however, most of the factors mentioned will be relevant at some time or another in your classes. Some methods may work for you, others may not. You could experiment with those suggestions that appeal to you and see whether they do work within your context.

CONDITIONS WITHIN THE SUBJECT MATTER

Special characteristics of specific subjects or disciplines will demand different skills and abilities of both learners and teachers so once again we will not be providing hard and fast rules for creating appropriate conditions, but rather general principles which you can apply when appropriate.

Activity:
Consider the discipline or subject that you teach. Can you represent the key features of that discipline and their relationships to each other in diagrammatic form? What types of learning are required of your students in order to master your subject?

Feedback:
If you were able to draw a diagram representing the basic structure of your subject you will now have before you your 'concept map' of your subject. **Concept mapping** has been described by Novak (1979) as a means for helping students to come to grips with the structure of topics they have to learn, it can also be used in assessment of student learning, but perhaps more importantly you

can use it to help you plan your teaching - if you have trouble making connections between key features of your subject imagine how difficult it will be for your students. Not only must students create their own networks for relating new topics to each other and to existing knowledge but most disciplines will also require learners to undertake a variety of types of learning. Gagne (Ch.3, 1974) has classified the main outcomes of learning as:

<u>Verbal information</u> - the basic store of facts and propositions.

<u>Intellectual skills</u> - consisting of the ability to discriminate among stimuli, to develop concepts which organise knowledge and enable the learner to identify a class of objects, and to learn rules which enable the learner to respond to concepts with appropriate actions. These intellectual skills build on each other in the sense that the simpler ones are prerequisites for the more complex.

<u>Cognitive strategies</u> - govern the learner's behaviour in dealing with the environment, the learner uses cognitive strategies to think about learning and to solve problems. As we have discussed earlier in this chapter cognitive strategies may be innate characteristics of the individual but they are also able to be learned and some educators have advocated their importance as educational goals in helping students 'learn how to learn' or 'learn to think' (Bruner, 1962).

<u>Attitudes</u> - a system of preferences which affect performance.

<u>Motor skills</u> - those manual or technical performances required in the application of what has been learned.

Using this classification you should reconsider the concept map of your subject and identify the various types of learning involved. Do they correspond with the types of learning you had originally identified? Have a close look at any discrepancies and make sure that you can apply the concepts presented to your subject area. It is probable that the emphasis may fall more heavily on some learning outcomes than others but it is also probable that all types of outcomes will be represented in your subject, at least to some extent.

Most learning theories acknowledge these different learning outcomes although emphasis differs and the strategies advocated for the achievement of each may also differ according to the philosophy and theoretical orientation of the educator. Some stress the sequential approach in which basic learning outcomes act as prerequisite building blocks for subsequent learning outcomes, for example children cannot learn to read until they can recognise and discriminate letters of the alphabet. Others see learning as a more idiosyncratic event in which learners incorporate knowledge and skills into existing cognitive structures in a sequence which is relevant to the task at hand, something like fitting pieces into a jigsaw puzzle and gradually building up a complete picture (Srinivasan, 1977). In fact both of these learning strategies are likely to be appropriate at different stages and in different contexts. The teacher's task is to ensure that students are sufficiently flexible to employ the most appropriate strategy for the learning objectives.

Problem-based learning and attention to the processes of learning which encourage active student involvement and application of learned knowledge and skills to novel situations are methods for increasing students' intellectual flexibility (for practical samples see Foley & Smilansky, Ch. 4, 1980, and subsequent chapters in this volume). Failure to promote this flexibility in students results in the all too familiar situation in which students learn facts, discriminations, concepts and principles which are stored in memory in a way which allows retrieval for examination purposes but which does not facilitate transfer to the practical situation. The problem is analogous to a filing system which is arranged according to date of receipt rather than function of documents. Retrieval of documents stored in the month of March is simple, as is recall of definitions learned in physiology lectures, however retrieval of documents required for the solution of a specific business problem will require a good deal of inefficient searching and trial and error, as would the solution of a clinical problem presenting as physiological disturbance. Knowledge which is not stored as part of a functional cognitive structure will not be efficiently used. Promotion of functional knowledge may be the biggest challenge facing nursing education especially as the location of nursing education transfers from hospital to college settings. According to Wong (1979) an understanding of the transfer of learning is critical to the success of the teaching-learning process and also critical to the improvement of nursing care.

Activity:
Refer to the first activity in this chapter in which you identified a personal learning experience which was either effective or ineffective. From your analysis of the reasons for the effectiveness of that experience and from your reading of this chapter work out some principles which describe the necessary conditions for learning knowledge, attitudes and skills.

Feedback:
   Once again there are no right or wrong answers in this activity. Conditions for learning will vary a great deal among cultures and teaching situations, however in general the following principles apply.

Conditions for learning knowledge
   For simplicity we will include Gagne's verbal information, intellectual skills and cognitive strategies under the general heading of knowledge. Knowledge is made up of the facts of the subject and the learners' ability to use those facts to think and solve problems.

1. Students must be presented with information in a form that they can understand. The most obvious example is that students must be familiar with the vocabulary and the concepts used. This is a common problem in nursing courses where many technical terms are needed. At a different level students must understand why they have to learn that information and how it can be made to fit with what they already know. In other words the information must be **relevant** to them.

2. <u>Students must be able to store information in
a way which facilitates its functional retrieval.</u>
If students are presented with information which is
totally unfamiliar they may be unable to relate it
to existing knowledge or to future tasks, they will
need advance organisers to help them classify the
new information, and they will need practical tasks
to encourage them to use the new information so
that it forms part of a useable cognitive
framework. Your own 'concept map' of the subject
might help you to make functional connections
explicit for the students. Helping students to
classify new information simplifies the learning
task because students can include the new
information under more general principles which are
already known, with the result that only specific
details need to be learned. For example, if we
classify a drug as belonging to the category of
beta-blockers then students who know about the
general characteristics of beta-blockers will need
to learn only those details such as toxicity levels
which are specific to that particular drug.
3. <u>Students must be able to use the information
they have learned to perform tasks or to solve
problems.</u> Unless students are given practice in
using the information they have learned it will be
quickly forgotten. To ensure that transfer to
clinical nursing is achieved it is important that
the opportunity for practice occurs in situations
as close as possible to situations they will
encounter in reality (see simulations in Chapter
6). But it isn't enough that we teach students to
solve a particular type of problem using particular
sets of information. Health care problems are not
predictable, patients will present with problems
which are difficult to classify, traditional
therapies may fail. No training course can ever
hope to cover all the possible situations the nurse
will confront. Students should therefore be
encouraged to strengthen and develop cognitive
strategies which will enable them to think on the
job, to create innovative solutions to unusual
problems and to generalise their professional and
personal experiences to responsive nursing
practice. Remember that there are individual
differences in students' preferred cognitive
strategies and in their aptitudes for learning
different types of information. Some students may

need more time, assistance and remedial work than others to achieve similar levels of competence.

4. <u>Students must have knowledge of the effectiveness of their use of information</u>. Feedback on the effectiveness of the cognitive strategies students use is essential if students are to maximise their potential. Feedback should be specific and diagnostic to enable students to rectify specific learning problems. It is not sufficient to say that the students' patient management plan is wrong, you must go through it with him or her and discuss both its strong points and its weak points to guide the students' processes of problem analysis. Discussions of process as well as content should be an integral part of learning as should be exercises in which students are able to judge their own performance and develop internal standards which are professionally appropriate.

<u>Conditions for learning attitudes</u>
        Attitudes may be defined as feelings, beliefs, values or preferences which influence the way the student behaves.

1. <u>Students cannot be taught attitudes in the same way that they are taught information or skills.</u> Because attitudes are involved with emotions they are personal and less accessible to the teacher. For this reason they are also difficult to assess, sources of external motivation are rarely effective in shaping desirable attitudes. It is highly desirable that nurses should have some particular attitudes which will assist them to gain the cooperation and trust of their patients and which will ensure that they conduct their professional tasks with responsibility. Teachers must therefore provide conditions in which favourable attitudes can develop. It is not sufficient to leave attitude formation to chance since students may well be exposed to quite powerful experiences which predispose to the formation of attitudes which are not desired learning outcomes (see Simpson, 1979).
2. <u>Students must be helped to recognise their existing attitudes</u>. Students come to nursing school with preconceived ideas about the role of a nurse,

the causes of illness, the feelings of patients, and many other aspects of health care. These ideas will be the products of their previous experiences and education. Some may be congruent with nursing practice and some may not. Before the incongruent attitudes can be changed the students must recognise them. Recognition of existing attitudes can be encouraged by discussion of controversial issues in class or by setting up activities in which students play roles (see Chapter 4).

3. <u>Students should be provided with new information which will challenge existing attitudes.</u> For example, as students come to know more about the physiology of certain diseases they may feel less worried about helping people with those diseases; as they become more skilled at specific tasks they may become less reticent about direct patient contact, as they become more familiar with nursing roles they may correct previous inaccurate perceptions.

4. <u>Students should be given the opportunity to test new attitudes.</u> Feedback is as important in the development of new attitudes as it is in the learning of knowledge or skills. For example a student may observe that a nurse who has a respectful attitude towards elderly patients is better able to gain their cooperation. Opportunities for work with elderly patients will then enable the student to try out aspects of behaviour that were observed. It is important to expose students to as many models of desired behaviour as possible. Opportunities for practice of modelled behaviour may be provided by role play, or class discussion prior to actual clinical contact but in all circumstances feedback is important so that the student realises how his or her attitudes influenced performance. Ideally, observation of videotape replay provides the most graphic feedback to students of their attitudes and behaviour.

Conditions for learning skills

Skills are performances that students learn through practice. In most cases they will be manual skills such as giving an injection or taking a blood pressure, but they may also be skills which involve communication, for example talking with a patient to explain a procedure.

1. <u>Students must know what it is they are expected to be able to do.</u> Students must observe someone demonstrating the skill effectively. Sometimes films are used to demonstrate skills which are difficult to set up in the classroom.

2. <u>Students must know how the skill is performed.</u> Most skills have a number of component subskills within them, each of which must be mastered before the student can perform the total skill. Each component subskill must therefore be demonstrated specifically so that the students' attention is drawn to specific aspects which contribute to effective performance. For example, adequate hand washing is a necessary component skill in applying a sterile dressing.

3. <u>Students must practise the skill.</u> Knowing how to perform the skill is not sufficient. There is a big difference between knowing how and actually doing well. In many cases practice may be difficult to obtain because it may involve risk or discomfort to patients. In such cases it is important to provide students with the opportunity to practise in a situation which resembles the real one closely but which does not carry any risks. This type of exercise is called a simulation. One example is the use of an orange to teach students how to give an injection. Another is for students to practise procedures on one another before they try them on people who are ill. As students begin to master the skill they may be progressively moved from simulation classes to real settings such as clinics. Practice in the real situation must be supervised until the teacher is confident that the skill has been mastered. Individual differences in aptitudes among students mean that students will not all achieve mastery at the same rate and flexibility should be built in to allow for longer practice periods and more feedback for those students who require it. It is unrealistic to assume that all will be equally skilled at the end of a course unless steps have been taken to diagnose those with a difficulty and provide remedial instruction.

4. <u>Students must receive feedback on their performance.</u> Practice alone is not sufficient for mastery of a skill, practice must be accompanied by knowledge of whether the performance is satisfactory. Feedback may be given by the teacher,

fellow students, patients or students themselves. Feedback must be specific and diagnostic - it must help the student identify specific aspects of performance which require further work. The ultimate aim of skill learning should be to transfer the students' dependence from the teacher's evaluation to personal or self-evaluation.

SUMMARY

Helping students learn is the primary role of the teacher. This chapter has examined some of the factors within the student, the learning context and the subject matter which influence student learning. Feasible strategies are available for the teacher to employ in each of those areas, all of those strategies depend on the teacher's willingness to become personally involved with students. Getting to know students' individual characteristics and needs, creating a climate of trust in which students can develop professional self-image and personal self-esteem, creating learning experiences which motivate, which allow for individual differences, active involvement, transfer and generalisation of learned information and skills, providing specific constructive feedback and encouraging growing self-reliance are essential parts of a nurse educator's role. The following chapters provide specific suggestions for creating those conditions in the variety of learning contexts found in schools of nursing.

Chapter 4.

MANAGING THE LEARNING SESSION

This chapter deals with the practical aspects of managing the learning session. In the previous chapters we have dealt with how you would decide what to teach and how you would decide which teaching methods to use. In this chapter we will look in more detail at some of those methods.

When you have finished this chapter you should be able to manage the following teaching methods effectively:
Lectures
Small group discussions
Role play and other simulations
Supervised clinical work
Independent learning.

In your use of all of these methods remember the conditions for learning which were discussed in Chapter 3. Your task as teacher is to try to create those conditions by skilful use of the methods described in this chapter. These methods have been chosen because they are the methods most commonly used by nursing instructors. You may already be familiar with, and skilled in, the use of some of the methods and you may wish to try integrating different aspects of the methods to increase the students' involvement with, and understanding of, what they need to learn. The references listed at the end of this chapter provide many interesting suggestions for innovations in teaching.

THE LECTURE

Planning a Lecture

In a previous chapter (Chapter 3) it was suggested that lectures are most useful when they are used to provide students with an overview of what they must know in a particular topic area. Lectures are best used to convey information which explains the relationships between detailed concepts in the topic and which is not readily available elsewhere.

Activity:
1. Select a topic about which you would normally give a lecture.
2. Write down a list of objectives for that lecture in terms of what you hope your students will gain from it.
3. List the key concepts or ideas which would form the main content of the lecture.
4. Plan the structure of your lecture, perhaps using a diagram to show the relationships between your key concepts, the sequence in which you will present them and the main examples you will use to expand your ideas.
5. Describe the teaching aids or resources you would use to help you make the lecture effective.
6. How will you check whether your objectives have been achieved?

Feedback for this activity will be arranged according to each of those tasks you have done in planning your lecture.

1. ## Selection of a Topic
Look at your topic again. Is your lecture the only formal teaching students will receive on that topic? Are the textbooks up to date in that area and are they easy for your students to understand? Is the topic one which has components of skills and attitudes as well as the knowledge you will be presenting in the lecture? Is the topic one which your students usually have difficulty with or is it fairly straightforward? Is the topic one which

generates a lot of student interest or do they usually find it dull or uninteresting?

2. Objectives for the Lecture

Your answers to the questions about your topic should help you to decide what your objectives for the lecture are. For example, if the topic is one which is not well covered by textbooks or other areas of teaching such as tutorials or clinical experiences your main objectives for the lecture may include the intention that students should be able to take a set of lecture notes which can serve as accurate reference material for their future learning (Information lecture).

If the topic is one which students usually find difficult to understand your objectives may include the intention that students will derive from the lecture a clearer picture of the main concepts and ideas and their relationships and thus develop a mental structure into which they can fit some of the more detailed aspects of the topic they will read about in their textbooks (Explanation lecture).

If the lecture is part of a larger set of experiences which include opportunities for learning skills and attitudes related to the topic, your objectives might be concerned with students gaining an overview of the topic and the relative importance of its component parts (Overview lecture).

If the topic is one which students usually find dull the objectives of the lecture should be concerned with students' motivation to learn the topic (Motivation lecture).

For convenience of reference each of these lectures has been given a name which appears in brackets at the end of the description. Of course, many lectures will contain elements of all or most of those objectives, but it is important nevertheless to decide what your objectives are so that you can plan a style and sequence of presentation that will be most effective in achieving them.

3. Content of the Lecture

Look at the key ideas and concepts you have decided to include in your lecture. Are they appropriate for your objectives? Do they motivate the student to want to learn the topic? Do they provide information which is not covered elsewhere or are they unnecessarily detailed, repeating essentially what is in the textbooks? Do they explain and put into context the relationship of the content of this lecture to the rest of the course?

4. Structure of the Lecture
    Bligh (1972) and Brown (1978) have both described a variety of lecture structures which may be used. Broadly, lectures fall into two main structure types, classical and problem-centred. The classical structure proceeds logically through information which is (usually) ordered from simple to complex, from normal to abnormal, from general principles to specific examples, leading the student progressively to an understanding of the overall topic through knowledge of its parts.

The problem-centred structure seems, at times, to do just the opposite, often providing examples of complex problems as the starting point and progressing through analysis of general principles, basic mechanisms and explanatory simpler information.

The structure you choose should depend on your personal preferences and on the objectives of the lecture. Teachers are usually more comfortable with the classical structure because it resembles the traditional explanatory structure of most disciplines and is the structure with which most teachers are familiar. It is also an easier structure for students to follow if their purpose is to take comprehensive notes from the lecture (Information lecture). The problem-centred structure on the other hand is a useful strategy for those lectures which are seen by students to be dull or even irrelevant (Motivation lecture). By providing clinical nursing problems as the basis for the information to be transmitted, the teacher helps the students to see why this information is necessary and how it fits into the job they are being trained for. Since the problem-centred lecture usually starts with a question it should also stimulate students' curiosity to follow the lecture through and arrive at the answer. A well planned problem-centred lecture can aid students to understand difficult concepts and their relationships to each other in a context which is

seen to be pertinent to the students' future role
(Explanation lecture, Overview lecture).
Problem-centred lectures, however, often result in
less comprehensive students' notes since the
emphasis is on the process of relating ideas to
problems and solutions rather than on presenting a
systematic body of information.

Whichever structure you have chosen the
general principles for presentation of the lecture
apply:

a) <u>Always start with a brief description of what
you intend to cover and the general structure
you intend to follow.</u> Remind students of
related information which they already know
and of the reasons why the topic of this
lecture is important for them.
Students are more motivated to learn when they
know what they are expected to learn and why
they need to learn it. Reminding students of
relevant previous learning helps them to grasp
the meaning of new information more easily.

b) <u>Use a series of major headings or subheadings</u>
on the board or in student handouts to sign-
post the direction in which you are heading
and to ensure that students can organize
their thinking and their notetaking.

c) <u>Use special techniques to emphasize the most
important points in the lecture.</u>
There are a number of ways to do this:
You can write key words or phrases on the
chalkboard
You can use audio-visual aids (See Chapter 6)
You can change the volume or expression of
your voice to awaken students' attention
You can repeat the important points for
emphasis
You can pause to ask the class a question
about the important points
You can use specific phrases to draw attention
such as 'Make sure you understand this'.

d)   <u>Summarize periodically the information you
     have covered.</u> This enables students to review
     what you have said and to ensure that they
     are following your line of evidence or
     information.

e)   <u>Encourage students to be actively involved
     during the lecture,</u> for example, give them a
     problem to solve or a question to answer.
     Active involvement serves two purposes:
     i) Students remember information better if
         they have to think about it as well as
         just copy it into their notes.
     ii) Research has shown that most students lose
         concentration, and their attention to the
         lecture starts to decrease after about
         15-20 minutes (Bligh, 1972, p. 73).
         Providing some activity after 20 minutes
         of the lecture serves to wake students up
         and to catch their attention again.
     (Some more ways of encouraging active
     participation in the lecture will be
     discussed in a following section.)

f)   <u>End the lecture by repeating the main points
     covered and by telling the students what the
     next lecture or teaching session will cover.</u>

5.   <u>Teaching Aids and Resources</u>
     Your objectives for the lecture should also
guide you in deciding what teaching aids and
resources you want to use. Details of resources are
dealt with in Chapter 6 so only brief mention will
be made here. Handouts are a useful resource in
'Information' lectures because they relieve the
student of some of the burden of notetaking.
Handouts may provide full information or an outline
of headings or main points. If your lecture is
predominantly an 'Explanation' lecture you may wish
to use a number of diagrams. Some teachers prefer
to draw diagrams on the chalkboard as they go along
but others find that prepared overhead
transparencies allow time to be saved and ensure
the clarity of the diagram. Diagrams can also be
provided as handouts to avoid transcription errors

which often result from hurried copying by students. If your lecture is an 'Overview' lecture or a 'Motivation' lecture you may find that use of colour photographs, motion pictures or video-cassette helps you to demonstrate aspects of the nurse's role which are difficult to describe but which explain the importance of the topic to be learned or demonstrate its skill and attitudinal components.

6. Check on Achievement of Objectives
    If you are an experienced lecturer you may be able to tell from audience non-verbal reaction whether your students are keeping up with the lecture or whether they have drifted off. Besides looking for informal cues such as an increase in the level of background conversation, or a cessation of notetaking, or an increased incidence of puzzled faces you can also arrange for formal gathering of feedback on students' understanding. You may leave time for questions during or after the lecture (particularly if your class is a small one). You may wish to ask students to fill out forms which provide feedback on specific aspects of your lecturing technique (See Chapter 8), you may rely on spot tests of lecture content in tutorials or, in the long term you may check performance on your lecture topics (in formal examinations). One useful method is to schedule follow-up tutorials on specific key points from the lecture and to invite students to attend for the purpose of clarifying their understanding. Such tutorials help both the teacher and the students to identify problem areas in teaching and learning.
    You may wish to undertake the following activity which provides practice in applying these principles of lecture planning.

Activity:
Choose another topic about which you may be asked to give a lecture. Write a lecture out-line for that topic following the guidelines suggested in the previous activity. Remember to define your objectives, outline your content, map out your structure and plan the resources and feedback mechanisms you will use.

Feedback for this activity is a lecture outline using contraceptive methods as an example topic.

LECTURE OUTLINE

Topic: Contraceptive methods.

Learners: Community Health Nurses

Purpose: The lecture is intended to provide an overview of the topic since a comprehensive and accurate account of the topic is provided in the textbook.

Objectives: After attending the lecture nurses should be able to
- describe the mechanisms of action of the four main types of contraceptives
- explain the indications and contra-indications for each which contribute to choice of method

Content, structure and resources:

Introduction: State and clarify the objectives for the lecture
Describe the nurses' future likely role in advising about contraception
Recall previous learning by asking nurses to write down a classification of the ways in which conception might be prevented

Key Points: 1. Conception may be prevented by preventing ovulation, fertilization or implantation.
Resource: Overhead transparency diagram of sites of action of main contraceptives.
2. Prevention of ovulation - provide handouts with graphs of ovulatory cycle - ask nurses to label graph curves with appropriate hormones. Describe mechanisms of action of hormonal contraceptives and the advantages and disadvantages.

Stop for questions
3. Prevention of fertilization - describe rhythm method - refer to handout of graph of ovulatory cycle.

Stop for discussion of advantages and disadvantages of rhythm method.

> Describe barrier methods, how do they work and advantages and disadvantages
> Resources: Samples &/or diagrams.

Summarise main points and allow a few minutes for questions

> 4. Prevention of implantation - Intra-uterine devices - how do they work, who are they suitable for? Resources: Samples and diagrams.

Clinical Problem:

> Present a brief case history and ask students to form small groups with those in adjacent seats to decide on the most appropriate contraceptive to recommend.
>
> Presentation of responses from 2 or 3 groups.
>
> Provide feedback to class on the correct choice and the reason for it. **Use this feedback to summarise the main points covered in the lecture.**

Closure: Tutorial to follow this lecture will deal with questions arising from the lecture. Advise students to read relevant chapters in the textbook.

<u>Outline of Handout to be used in Lecture:</u>

---

1. Objectives for the lecture

2. Use the following questions as headings with space for students' notes:
   . How do the hormonal contraceptives work?
   . What is the basis of the rhythm method?

. What are the most reliable barrier contraceptives?
. What are the main indications for the use of IUD?

3. Graph of ovulatory cycle - labelling to be completed by students

4. Summary list of main contra-indications to use of each of the contraceptives described.

In Summary, your lecture outline may be quite different from the one suggested here. That does not matter. The important thing is to remember the basic principles:

Introduction	**- To set objectives** **- To motivate** **- To remind them of other related knowledge**
Logical organization	**- Use lists of key points, handouts**
Emphasise main points	**- Use audio-visual aids, questions, repetition**
Student participation	**- Buzz groups, question time, incomplete handouts**
Summarise	**- At the end of each section** **At the end of the lecture**
Closure	**- Refer to other classes plus follow-up activities** **Check their understanding**

Presenting a Lecture

Of course, knowing how to plan a lecture is only half of the story. Even a well planned lecture will suffer from poor presentation by the lecturer. Skills in presentation can only be gained by practice and feedback on performance. We will be dealing with evaluation of teaching skills in Chapter 8, but in the meantime you might like to consider some informal ways of seeking feedback on your lecturing skills. You could, if you have the resources, request that your lectures be videotaped so that you can get a student's eye view of yourself, or if that is not possible you may make an audiotape of your lectures so that you can at least hear what your lecture sounded like. This is an excellent way of finding out how well you have structured your presentation and your explanations. Another option is to develop a reciprocal arrangement with a trusted fellow teacher who can observe your lectures and also be observed by you for the purposes of constructive suggestions for improvement. Start by asking for feedback on areas of your teaching which concern you and gradually build up to those areas such as personal mannerisms, which may be more personally threatening.

As you become more comfortable with some of the basic suggestions presented in this book you may wish to experiment with different methods of involving students or with different ways of presenting material or using audio-visual aids. Many helpful suggestions can be found in Quinn (1980), Brown (1978), Powell (1973), and Bligh, (1972).

SMALL GROUP DISCUSSION

In this section of the chapter we will be looking at small groups used as a method for increasing student discussion. For our purposes a small group will be defined as a group of less than fifteen people who are meeting for an educational purpose. There are many different ways in which learning in small groups may be encouraged, The way that you plan and conduct small group learning should be determined by two considerations:

i) What you are trying to achieve - your objectives for the session.

ii) What you and your students are comfortable with.

Many teachers complain that their students will not participate in group discussion so that teachers might just as well give a lecture to a large group. The following activities and suggestions are intended to help you overcome this problem and to develop ways for gaining maximum benefit from small group learning sessions.

The first consideration is to decide what purposes small group learning is best suited for.

Activity:
What types of learning can be achieved more effectively in small groups than in other ways? Make a list of the teaching situations in which you would choose to use a small group rather than another type of learning situation.

Feedback:

Small group sessions are useful for:
1. **Involving students as active participants in the learning task, rather than passive listeners.**
2. **Developing skills in teamwork and cooperation.**
3. **Developing manual, or physical or communication skills through practice and feedback from the teacher and other students.**
4. **Providing practice in applying knowledge to solving problems individually or as a member of a group.**
5. **Encouraging students to try out new attitudes and ideas with a group of their peers.**
6. **Providing opportunities for students to have close contact with a teacher and to check out their understanding.**

You may also have thought of other purposes, but if you found it difficult to answer the questions in this activity you should refer back to Chapter 3. The important thing to remember about the purposes of small group learning is that the interaction among members of the group is the critical event. Learning how to approach and solve problems, developing skills, and forming attitudes can be achieved in small groups because **the members of the group can help and stimulate each other** to work through whatever the learning task is.

The help and support that group members can provide for each other may not be present in the initial stages of group work, but if the teacher is sensitive and able to help this climate of support to develop, then productive, cooperative relationships usually result. In fact, one of the most important purposes of group work is to help students develop skills in teamwork. Such skills will be important in the performance of their clinical tasks.

Activity:
Next time that you are involved in a group discussion take notice of what is happening in the group. The group you observe may be a learning group or an informal meeting for social or administrative purposes. To help you in your observations of the group you may like to keep the following questions in mind:
Who spoke first?
Who seemed to be the 'leader' of the group - what was that person doing which gave you the impression that he or she was the leader?
Who talks to whom?
What was the emotional climate in the group like - were people happy, productive, bored, aggressive? What were the factors contributing to that climate?
Are there any patterns which emerge in the behaviour of the members of the group?
From your observations of the group can you draw any conclusions about factors which influence the effectiveness of discussion in groups?

Feedback:
There are many excellent books available which deal with small group dynamics in general (for example see Applbaum et al.,1974; McLeish et al., 1973 and Abercrombie, 1979) and in nursing in particular (for example see Quinn, 1980, de Tornyay, 1971). Some of the main points which bear on the function of small discussion groups are summarised below.

Physical Environment
Small group function is facilitated by an environment which allows a degree of relaxation by participants. If it is possible to provide comfortable chairs, tea or coffee making facilities and pleasant, private surroundings so much the better. Most teachers however will have to make do with standard teaching accommodation, but the crucial point to remember is that if you want students to talk to each other then seating must be arranged so that they can comfortably see each other.
The most effective seating arrangement for a discussion group is to have all participants seated so that they are facing each other. Usually this is achieved by placing seats in a circle or an oval. If the group's task will require students to do some writing then a table can be placed in the centre. This sort of arrangement can also be achieved in a traditional science laboratory without too much trouble by arrangement of seats around the end and sides of a laboratory bench. The same effect can also be achieved (although not so comfortably) in an ordinary lecture theatre by asking students to turn sideways in their seats to talk with students in the row behind, or in front. Whenever possible if you, the teacher, are to take part in the discussion you should be seated in the circle too. If the teacher sits apart from the group then students will automatically assume the role they have in a lecture and expect the teacher to do all of the talking. Which brings us to a consideration of the role of the teacher in small group discussion.

The Role of the Teacher
There are no hard and fast rules for the role the teacher will play in the group. Obviously the

teacher's role will vary with the objectives of the discussion and with the type of students who are being taught. The main thing to remember is that it is an inefficient use of time if the members of a small group spend their time listening to what the teacher has to say, because this is in effect, a lecture which might just as easily be given to a large group of students. Of course, for some types of learning objectives the teacher will have a major role to play, perhaps by demonstrating a particular clinical skill or in guiding students through difficult material towards an understanding of the main concepts. However, even though the teacher has a major role the key to learning lies in the students' ability to participate in practice of the skill or in thinking through the difficult aspects of a problem. For other types of learning objectives it may be more appropriate for the teacher to attempt to be an equal member of the group, allowing other group members to take leadership where appropriate. This approach is most appropriate where the intention is to stimulate students to examine issues, attitudes or feelings in areas in which expertise is less important than personal experience. Depending on the maturity of the group the teacher may find it necessary to play an intermediate role, that of a facilitator - a friendly guide who keeps a watchful eye on the process of the group and intervenes with sensitivity to ensure that objectives are achieved and a positive climate maintained in the group.

The Role of the Students

Small group discussion offers the students the chance to learn by doing. Students must therefore come to the group prepared to work. Since many students' previous educational experiences have accustomed them to a fairly passive approach to learning, students do not always find it easy to adapt to a learning situation in which they must take responsibility for what happens during their time together with the teacher. Sometimes they express impatience with the process of group discussion and insist that they would learn more if the teacher would just tell them what it is that they are supposed to know. In some cases previous bad experiences of small group learning may have resulted in frustration or withdrawal from

91

participation. Some of these negative reactions to small group work can be forestalled by the teacher if he or she is aware of the dynamics of group interaction and of approaches which provide structure where necessary, and freedom where desirable in order to minimise frustration and maximise satisfaction and productivity.

Experts in the behaviour of people in groups state that all groups go through six broad stages of development. These stages are said to occur in some form regardless of the task of the group, or the type of participants, or the duration of the group's meeting.

Stage 1:   Getting to know each other
In this stage little work is done and group members talk to each other on a fairly superficial level while they become comfortable with each other. The teacher can help students through this stage by creating a warm friendly atmosphere and by inviting students to talk with each other informally before they begin the task.

Stage 2 :   Defining the purpose of the meeting
In this stage group members attempt to sort out the purpose of the meeting, they sometimes experience a lack of direction or frustration and may become impatient. The teacher can help here by guiding discussion in useful directions or by helping students to clarify what they expect to achieve in the group.

Stage 3 :   Establishing working rules and norms for behaviour
In this stage ground rules are established. Group members may decide on a strategy for achieving the task, or an order of business to attend to.

Stage 4 :   Active contribution
By this stage group members have a commitment to the group and its task. Cooperation increases and decisions are made (explicitly or implicitly) about whom will do what and when to achieve the task.

Stage 5 :   A sense of accomplishment
              Members undertake effective group
              work to complete their task. At this
              stage group members may feel pleased
              with themselves and the mood of the
              group is usually a positive one.

Stage 6 :   The end of the task
              Group members 'wind down' from the
              task and carry out final jobs
              associated with it. The coherence of
              the group begins to break down.

Of course some of these stages will assume more prominence than others according to the tasks or objectives of the group. For example a group which is meeting for the main purpose of learning how to pass a naso-gastric tube will spend most of its time and energy in stages 4 and 5. On the other hand a group which has as its objective the development of a nursing plan for a given patient case may need to spend considerable time in stages 2 and 3 before they can hope to be productive in stages 4 and 5. Stage 1 is essential for all groups where the students and the teacher have not worked together before.

Occasionally a group may have more difficulty in one or other stage, particularly in stages 2 and 3. If you are aware that these are normal phases that groups pass through then you will be able to help resolve some of the conflicts so that the group can move on to productive activity. As students become more experienced at working in groups they may also begin to take facilitatory roles in some of the more problematic stages. Since one of the aims of group discussion is to improve students' ability to work together they should be encouraged to understand the processes of the group and to accept responsibility for ensuring its effective function.

When the members of a group work together for a period of time it may also be possible to observe certain roles emerging. You may have noted these roles in your observations of a group. In general the roles fall into two categories - roles associated with the task and roles associated with the social maintenance of the group. Task roles may include initiating action, doing routine chores, gathering information, assigning jobs, drawing group members back to the task, keeping discussion on the track and evaluating group output. Social roles may include keeping interpersonal relations pleasant, handling conflict, providing encouragement, relieving tension through humour, giving silent members a chance to be heard, and observing and commenting on the process of the group. All of these roles may of course be filled by the experienced teacher, however one of the objectives of any small group learning session should be to encourage students to develop skills in some of those roles themselves, since those skills will be transferable to their professional work on the wards and in the community.

Now that we have considered some of the factors which influence the way learning groups work, it may be useful to turn to a consideration of some of those factors which sometimes impede the function of the group.

Activity:
Think back to the group that you observed or to some other group in which you have recently participated as teacher or learner. What were some of the problems which arose in the process of the group discussion and what could the group facilitator or teacher have done to avoid those problems?

Feedback :   **Problems for the group leader**

1. Teachers are often tempted to take over the group and do most of the talking, or, in the case of skill learning, do most of the work.

Students may be willing for this to happen because it saves them from having to work. One of the hardest things for a teacher to learn is to tolerate silence in the learning group. Sometimes a period of silence means that people are thinking and will soon share their thoughts with the rest of the group - if the teacher hurries in to fill the gap the students will not be able to take full advantage of the group activity. Similarly, if the teacher spends all the time demonstrating a

94

particular skill students will have no opportunity to do it themselves. Watching is not a substitute for doing.

2. Talkative students may dominate the group making it difficult for quiet or shy students to enter the discussion.

Teachers must develop tactful ways to control dominant students and encourage quiet students. This may be done by gentle probing such as (to a quiet student): 'What do you think about that?' or 'Is that the way you think it should be done?' A dominant group member can sometimes be given tasks to do which will occupy her and direct her energy in a productive way. She could for example be made responsible for writing the group's findings on the board. Or the teacher can tactfully direct questions elsewhere, for example (to dominant student): 'So that's what you have experienced with this problem in your clinic'; and (to the rest of group): 'Have the rest of you had any other sorts of experiences?'

3. Group discussion may become side-tracked from the main purposes of the discussion.

To some extent this may be a good thing. Groups should be able to talk about interesting side issues which crop up. These discussions will also contribute to their learning. However you will have to judge when the side issues are taking too much time away from the main object of the discussion. You can get the group back onto the track by saying something like: "That's an interesting point which we could look at later but let's get back to the main point and see what we should do about it first". Sometimes, as the group begins to function better some of your students may adopt these "facilitator roles" as well and should be encouraged to do so.

4. Sometimes the group discussion may become nothing more than a question and answer session where you ask questions or respond to students' questions.

This is a popular format often seen in small group sessions after a lecture and it does have a

95

place for clarifying understanding. However it may be timewasting for some students who are not involved in the discussions. A better way is to ask students for their questions at the beginning and then to set the group the task of answering them. You might act as an extra resource if necessary. Students then benefit not only from having their questions answered but from having to work out and deliver explanations to each other. Explaining is an excellent test and reinforcer of learning.

5.   Sometimes the teacher does not organise the time well enough to allow everyone to benefit from the session.

For example if the group members are expected to learn a skill the session should be organised so that all members have an opportunity for some practice and feedback on their performance.

6.   Sometimes the discussion enters areas in which neither the teacher nor the students has the knowledge or skills to proceed productively.

Some teachers find this threatening and tend to direct students towards other more comfortable areas, resulting in the students feeling frustrated and sometimes losing trust or confidence in the teacher. This situation may be avoided by establishing norms or ground rules early in the discussion which clarify your role as a resource for the group rather than as an expert with all of the answers. As a resource you should be able to help the students to determine where they can find the information or skills that are lacking.

In summary, an effective group leader should plan activities which will achieve the learning objectives and encourage student interaction. Productive group discussion cannot be left to 'just happen'. The teacher or group leader and the students must know what the aim of the discussion or activity is and the teacher must be prepared to take action when necessary to create conditions which will be best for the group task. Sometimes this means suggesting an activity, or providing information or helping students to overcome personal differences and sometimes it means having the skill, the patience and the trust to leave students to their own devices at the appropriate time.

Some excellent suggestions for maximising group effectiveness can be found in articles by Smallegan (1982) and Lee (1978a,b,c&d). Detailed suggestions for specific activities in specific topics are also provided in subsequent chapters in this book.

Planning a Small Group Session

Activity:
Now that you have some new ideas about making groups work it will be helpful if you put them into practice to see how well they work with your subject and your students. Plan a small group session for a topic that you teach. Pay particular attention to the following:
1. How will you introduce the topic?
2. How will you encourage participation by group members?
3. How will you finish off the discussion or activity?

Feedback:
Needless to say that you should begin your planning by deciding what the objectives of the learning session are. Don't forget that since you are using a small group for the topic you should try to include objectives which make use of the capacity for practice, interaction and feedback. In other words you should use the small group as an opportunity for attitudes and skill learning as well as the acquisition of knowledge. Since you may not always have complete control over the direction in which students take the discussion you should give careful thought to the **key areas** or **key questions** which you would like to be addressed by the group. If their discussions take them into those areas well and good, if not you can be prepared to judiciously insert probing or leading questions which will bring those key issues to the fore.

Decide on the level of autonomy you wish the group to have and therefore on the level of control

97

you wish to exert over the activities of the group. If you intend to maintain a low profile it will be particularly important for you to provide an introduction to the topic which will allow the students to define its scope and direction without having to guess what you want them to do.

The following suggestions are an incomplete list of strategies you may use for getting the group started and keeping it going.

Starting the Group Discussion

The way you start the discussion should motivate students to want to talk about the topic or undertake the task.

- Use a case study, film or story to focus students on the topic and help them to see its relevance to the tasks of the nurse.
- Show enthusiasm for the topic and an interest in tackling the problem or procedure yourself.
- Try to choose a problem or task that the students see as important - you might want to involve them in the choice of specific topics or tasks to be undertaken.
- Clearly define the problem or topic to be addressed and the nature of the task confronting the group. Tell them the objectives or enlist their aid in defining or modifying the objectives.

Encouraging Group Participation

- Arrange seating in such a way that group members can freely talk to each other.
- Try to ensure that group members are prepared for the discussion by notifying them of the topic in advance, prescribing prior activities or prereading assignments.
- Resist the temptation to talk too much and provide all the answers. Given enough time to become comfortable and to think, most group members find that they can contribute usefully to each other's knowledge and skills.
- Be aware of the stages that groups pass through and be prepared to help the group through difficult phases. Use gently probing questions which focus the discussion and encourage quieter group members to speak.

- Be aware of the various roles that members of the group are assuming, and of the ways in which they participate, and be prepared to help them to learn effective ways to contribute to the discussion or task.

Finishing off the Discussion
- Warn students 10 minutes before the end of time so that they can come to some conclusions or closure in their discussion or task.
- Summarise or encourage the students to summarise the discussion and highlight the main points discussed and the main achievements in relation to the objectives.
- Review the work which still needs to be done and set the task for the next meeting.

Specific strategies for encouraging group discussion are many. One of the most relevant and effective strategies in use in nurse education is the role play.

ROLE PLAY

One method which is commonly used in small groups in nurse education is role play (for example see Schweer, 1972). Role play is a method in which students take the roles of participants in a situation. The general aim of role play is to enable students to experience situations and learn to deal with them before they meet them in real life.

Purposes of Role Play

Activity:
You may have used role play or considered using it in your teaching. Make a list of the purposes or learning objectives which role play can help nursing students achieve.

Feedback:

The main purpose of role play is to enable students to practise skills or to experience their own and others' reactions to particular situations they will face in nursing practice. Undoubtedly, these same skills and reactions can be encountered in real life situations such as ward or community work, however, nursing practice deals with sensitive issues and situations which may involve risk to patients. Opportunities to practise in simulated or life-like situations are needed before students can apply their skills in caring for real patients or solving real problems. Specific purposes for which role play is often used include the following:

1. Learning communication skills, for example interviewing a patient or relatives.
2. Learning procedural skills, for example taking blood pressure or assisting in the operating theatre.
3. Learning about relationships between people, for example the members of the health team and the factors which assist or impede their ability to work together.
4. Exploring emotions involved in certain types of situation or with certain types of behaviour, for example caring for terminally ill patients, sick children and their families.
5. Trying out new behaviour, skills or attitudes in situations which resemble reality but which allow for feedback and no risks to the patient or the student.

An important aspect of the role play is that even though players are acting a role they should be free to express their own reactions and feelings spontaneously within that role. Players do not rehearse parts or learn scripts but make up their own responses within the general scenario, as the role play goes on. People vary in their ability to put themselves into a role but with support, encouragement and an informal relaxed atmosphere generated in a group who are used to working together, most students find that they can participate to some extent. Some roles generate significant reactions within some players and some groups, so a vital component of all role play should be the 'deroling' which follows. In this deroling players are given an opportunity to discuss their feelings and reactions to the role and to differentiate between their real feelings and those that were only a part of the role. It is the teacher's responsibility to ensure that the discussion following the role play contributes to the students' achievement of the learning objectives, and provides an opportunity for resolution or follow up of any problems that may have surfaced in the individual or the group.

Planning and conducting a Role Play

Successful role plays don't just happen they have to be planned. The degree of guidance which might be given to players and the group will depend to a large extent on the objectives of the session and on the level of experience of the group. However, the basic steps to be followed in planning a role play remain fairly constant.

1.   Set objectives for the role play

Prepare the students by telling them what the role play is supposed to achieve in general terms. Make sure that the students have enough background knowledge and that they can relate the role play to familiar experiences.

Example of objectives for a role play.
i)   To develop skills in providing medication instructions to patients on discharge from hospital.
ii)   To identify the difficulties inherent in transferring an elderly patient from the hospital environment to self care when several medications are necessary.
iii)   To explore the responsibilities of the patient, the doctor, the nurse and the family in ensuring optimal care.
iv)   To experience the feelings of an elderly patient who is being discharged from hospital on a new treatment regimen.

2.   Prepare a scenario

The scenario is a brief outline of the situation

which provides the setting, the problem or situation involved and the motives of the players. Each player is told something of his or her own motives but not of the motives of the other players (as is usually the case in real life situations). You must provide enough detail to get the players started but not so much that the players have no room to express their own emotions and reactions in the roles.

Example of a scenario
Setting
By the bedside. An 83 year old man is being discharged from hospital after three weeks as an inpatient undergoing treatment for digitalis intoxication, cardiac arrhythmia and congestive cardiac failure. His dosage of digitalis has been halved, he is taking a stronger diuretic and some potassium supplements and vitamin supplements at various times of the day. He understands from hearing medical students talk about his case that he was ill because he had been taking too high a dose of his heart tablets before coming into hospital. He lives in a self-contained flat behind his daughter's house but is alone most of the day because his daughter's family go to work and school.

Players
The old man - you are slightly deaf. You are afraid that your daughter's family don't want you back because you are a burden to them. You do not understand why you have to take all of these new tablets especially since you understand that your recent illness was caused by too much of one of them. You don't like to ask the doctors too many questions because they always seem to be busy so you have asked the nurse to explain what tablets should be taken and when you can stop taking them.

The nurse - You are a junior nurse and you are surprised that the patient is asking about his medications. You assumed that it was the doctor's responsibility to explain this to the patient, in any case you have not been very involved with this patient's management and

are not sure of the reasons for his change
of medication. You decide to talk to the
patient's daughter when she comes to collect
him because the old man is a little deaf and
you don't have too much time to spend
explaining. The doctor is in the clinic and
unable to come to the ward. The head nurse has
to provide a report on your work and you are
reluctant to reveal that you do not know how
to handle the situation.

The daughter - You are worried because your
father almost died before he came into
hospital and you are afraid that he will
become ill at home again and that you won't be
able to look after him. You haven't seen his
doctor in the hospital because he is usually
not around at visiting hours but you seek
reassurance from the nurse who seems to be
looking after your father.

The head nurse - You are aware of the
situation and have decided to see how the
nurse handles the situation before stepping in
to help her out. You intend to discuss the
problem with her later and point out how she
could improve her skills in this area.

3.   **Assign roles**

Players should volunteer to take part. Other group
members should act as observers to take note of
interesting events in the role play for discussion
afterward. While players are taking a few minutes
to prepare for their roles, observers could be
discussing the issues or points that should be
looked out for in that scenario with those
particular objectives. Alternatively, you can
provide the observers with a list of things to
watch for - this list will depend on the objectives
of the session.

4.   **Carry out the role play**

Players should respond spontaneously to each other
for as long as the activity is important and
relevant. Take care to stop the role play before it
becomes boring or before so much happens that you

103

won't be able to discuss it all. Of course you should be sensitive to what is happening in the role play and only stop it when it gets to a natural break in the interactions.

If you have video tape equipment it is very helpful to record the role play so that it can be referred to during the following discussion.

5.   Follow-up discussion

The purpose of this discussion is to allow students to talk about, understand, and receive feedback on the experience they have just had.

Players should try to describe their view of what happened and the reactions engendered in themselves and other players. These views should then be compared with information gathered by the observers. Discussion should try to identify the patterns in relationships and the causes and effects of the events in the role play and then transfer these patterns to relevant real life experiences. The role play should always be tied back into the real situation in which students will eventually find themselves.

Activity:
Identify a situation in your teaching area which might be effectively illustrated by a role play.
Write a scenario for the role play and try it out with your students.

Feedback:
Use the following checklist to assess how effective your role play was

	Yes	No
Were the objectives clear to participants at the beginning?	...	...
Was the scenario good enough to promote the behaviour you wanted to demonstrate?	...	...

	Yes	No
Were the players able to play their roles?	...	...
Were the players able to describe their experiences and attitudes to the group?	...	...
Did students gain appropriate feedback on their skills or attitudes?	...	...
Did the observers observe relevant information and report it to the group?	...	...
Was the group able to draw some conclusions about the causes and effects of the behaviours demonstrated in the role play?	...	...
Were the objectives of the role play achieved?	...	...
Did the group enjoy the experience and find it worthwhile?	...	...

If your answers to any of these questions were 'no' then you should reread the section on role play and check each part of your role play exercise to see where you could improve it. Feedback from students or colleagues who participated in the role play should help you here.

Don't give up if you have one unsuccessful experience - role play is a method which improves with practice for both teacher and students.

CLINICAL LEARNING

A broad definition of clinical learning is 'learning which occurs in settings similar to the ones in which the student will eventually work.'
Adopting this broader definition allows us to shift the focus from purely bedside activities (the traditional meaning of the word clinical) to the

105

broader range of activities the nurse will find herself involved in. These other activities include community services of various kinds.

Different countries or even institutions within countries have evolved different systems for providing clinical training. The differences lie in the extent to which the nursing student is seen solely as a student,or as a working nurse or as a combination of both. However, whatever the primary organisation of nursing education the basic skills required by the nurse are the same and the learning activities required for the development of those skills are ultimately very similar regardless of setting. One problem that most systems seem to have in common is the difficulty of helping students make the transition from classroom to clinic or ward and from knowledge acquisition to application of that knowledge in the solution of clinical problems. Problems may be further compounded by conflicts which arise between the trainee nurse's educational and service roles and the expectations of clinical educators and supervisors in relation to those roles. Good communication between school-based nurse educators, clinical supervisors and students is a vital component of clinical learning and should be foremost in mind when the objectives and methods of clinical learning are being considered.

Aims of Clinical Education

Activity:
Clinical education is vital for the preparation of professional nurses who can function competently and independently in a diversity of nursing situations. Make a list of the main aims of clinical education.

Feedback:
Much has been written about the aims of clinical education (for examples see Infante, 1975, Hinchliff, 1979, Kilmon et al, 1980). The general aims for clinical education seem to fall into five main areas:
1. To help students to learn skills they will

need as nurses and to gain an understanding of
the principles underlying those skills.

2. To help students learn to deal with situations
    and people they will meet in the nursing role.
3. To provide students with supervised practice
    in applying their factual knowledge and
    learned skills to the solution of real
    problems in the practical situation.
4. To help students to understand the jobs they
    are learning to do and to gain confidence in
    their own abilities to carry out their role.
    To guide the student in the transition from
    student to independent professional.
5. To enable students to work with senior
    practitioners who can model appropriate
    behaviour and attitudes, and to expose
    students to experiences which will help to
    shape their attitudes in desirable directions.

These are the purposes for which clinical
education can be used, however, unless the clinical
experience is planned with these explicit aims in
mind it can be a frustrating experience which does
not achieve its full potential.

Effective Clinical Education

Activity:
Think of the clinical education that you have
experienced, either as a student or teacher.
From your own experience identify the problems
which can arise in clinical work and therefore
the characteristics of effective clinical
experiences which avoid those problems.

Feedback:
The problems most commonly identified include
the following:
-   Clinical experiences are sometimes difficult
    to arrange because the clinical setting is
    also a service setting and full-time staff are
    usually concerned with their patient care
    responsibilities. Students may either be
    unwelcome because they 'just get in the way',
    or conversely students may be welcome as an

107

extra pair of hands rather than a learner with learning needs to be met.

- Clinical supervisors may not be fully aware of the objectives of the placement or of the background knowledge and skills that students have when they arrive. In situations in which students are needed to fulfil service roles they may even be assigned to clinical areas in which they have had no background learning, for example Paediatrics. In such cases students will have little opportunity to achieve the objectives for which the placement was intended.

- Students themselves may be ignorant of the objectives or specific purposes of the placement and therefore unable to properly direct their own learning efforts. They may be uncomfortable in the clinical setting and have uncertainties about their roles and others' expectations of them.

- Supervisors may misuse the unique learning opportunities provided by clinical education by teaching students in the same way as they would in the classroom. For example, handovers at report time may become mini-lectures, instead of an opportunity for the students to practise giving a report and getting feedback about the care given to patients assigned to them.

- Assessing the students' learning in clinical work is difficult because much of the learning which takes place is difficult to observe or measure objectively. The usual written tests will not adequately assess clinical skills and attitudes.

- In the clinical situation the presence of a patient may complicate the teaching and learning process since both teachers and students must take care to ensure that they do not cause the patient undue discomfort or concern.

- In some organisational frameworks for clinical teaching the respective roles of school-based nurse educators and service-based clinical supervisors may give rise to uncertainties over role definition and acceptance of responsibility for various aspects of training. If clear lines of communication and accountability for the student are not defined the student becomes the proverbial 'meat in the sandwich' and may miss many valuable opportunities for guidance and feedback.

How can these problems and others which you may have identified be overcome?

Firstly, it is important that clear objectives for each clinical experience be identified and shared with students and clinical staff. These objectives should refer not only to the knowledge, skills and attitudes that the students should gain but also to the level to which the student should be expected to perform. Pascasio (1975) has classified three levels of clinical learning experiences:

a) an initial introduction to the 'real' health care world and roles,
b) reinforcement through practice under supervision,
c) internship in which nurses function as health professionals in the service role.

Most clinical education falls into categories a) and b) with c) coming later in the students' course of study when a reasonable level of competence has been achieved to the satisfaction of both students and teachers.

Initial introduction to the real health care world.
This initial introduction can take the form of tutorials in which students and teacher work through case studies of patient problems and their solution, role plays in which simulated situations are encountered and dealt with, and class laboratories where various patient simulations are available for demonstration of skills and procedures. Effective simulations can be achieved by students working with each other, alternately playing the part of patients and nurse.

Frequently, as part of these introductory experiences the teacher will be called upon to demonstrate skills or techniques. Inexperienced teachers sometimes fall into the trap of assuming that demonstration is sufficient to ensure that students know how to proceed with practising the skill. This is not necessarily so. There are three steps in a successful demonstration: demonstration, followed by supervised practice of the components of the task, followed by return demonstration in which the students demonstrate that they are able to integrate the components into performance of the task. It is worth taking a little time out here to look at the **characteristics of an effective demonstration.** The following checklist may be useful if you have to plan demonstrations from time to time:

1. What are the purposes or objectives of your demonstration?

    If your objectives require students to be able to perform the task you are demonstrating then you must also provide opportunities for practise and feedback.

2. What can you do to increase the students' involvement in the demonstration?

    Almost by definition a demonstration causes the audience to be passive. Learners learn better when they are actively involved. You should therefore plan your demonstration so that students are required to become involved in it in some way rather than to just watch. Ask some students to help, some to act as observers, provide written handouts and questions to guide students' thinking and observations, stop the demonstration at suitable points for questions and discussion and make sure that every student has a good view of what is happening.

3. What are the main points you want to make in the demonstration?

    Begin the demonstration by telling students briefly what you are about to do and summarise the main points they should watch for. You could choose some of the students to note down their observations at those key points and you should also point these out as they occur. By providing such a 'road map' through the demonstration you can ensure that students do not get lost in the technical details which might be likely to distract their attention.

At the end of the demonstration ask the students to summarise the lessons learned.

4. What resources will you require to carry out the demonstration?

Obviously you will assemble and check all the necessary technical equipment or materials for your demonstration beforehand. It is also worth thinking about whether any additional resources such as diagrams or handouts will help the students to get the most benefit from the demonstration. For example you could provide an observation checklist which requires the students to fill in their observations against certain questions or headings on the sheet.

5. Is the relevance of the demonstration clear?

Since demonstrations can be quite complex and time-consuming you should be sure that the demonstration is actually necessary for the achievement of your objectives. You should also make sure that students understand the relevance of the demonstration to what they are learning to do. Otherwise they may find it confusing or boring.

6. Have you provided opportunities for supervised practice and return demonstration?

Once you are satisfied with the students' level of skill and understanding of the basic principles applied to clinical practice then the students can be moved on through the next level of clinical education which is practice under supervision in a real setting, most often, the ward or community centre.

Practice under Supervision. Transition from classroom or simulated nursing laboratory into the real setting is the point at which many of the previously mentioned problems in clinical education arise. Some of those problems can be avoided by

111

adequate prior planning and preparation of both students and clinical staff and some of them can be avoided by improving knowledge and practice of the supervision role.

Preparation and planning

-   To avoid the problem of students 'getting in the way' or being unwelcome in the clinical setting it is necessary to prepare the students well. Make sure that they understand the functions and organisation of the ward or clinic and their place within those functions. This may have to be negotiated with clinical staff beforehand. Pascasio (1975) has outlined some of the processes of effective negotiation for use of clinical facilities.
-   Supervisors and clinical teachers should be involved in the planning of objectives for clinical placements and should be consulted on the most appropriate tasks for the students. Regular planning or review sessions between placement supervisors and school-based teachers are a useful source of feedback to both groups on how well the curriculum is preparing the students for their jobs.

Student supervision and activities

-   One of the biggest potential advantages of clinical education is that it provides students with the opportunity to plan their own learning which will allow them to follow their own interests as well as achieving the stated learning objectives. To allow this to happen the placement must give enough flexibility to allow individual student projects but also enough structure and guidance to ensure that students don't become 'lost' in the complexity of the situation. For example, students should be assigned to a supervisor or adviser with whom they can discuss their problems and what they have learnt. Regular sessions where groups of students and other staff can share their experiences in the placement may also be helpful. It is essential that opportunities be provided, in either simulated or low patient risk situations for the students to have the freedom to observe, plan, test and evaluate their own activities. The teacher must be able to stand back and allow the students to investigate and practice and discover things for themselves. The temptation to explain everything must be resisted in favour of leaving some unknowns for the students to discover for themselves (Infante, 1975).

- Clinical training offers students the opportunity to practise the roles for which they are training. To help them to do this students need a clear idea of their roles and their relationships with other members of the health care team.

One way to achieve this is to give students specific jobs to do, for example, taking histories of new patients or assisting in immunisation programs. Of course it is important that the students' tasks are appropriate to the objectives of the placement.

- Clinical teachers and supervisors may need to be trained to make the best educational use of the placement. Research into effective clinical teaching suggests that:

a) Active student participation should be encouraged.

Students gain more from practising clinical or practical skills and getting feedback from the teacher than they gain from merely watching the teacher performing.

One way to achieve this is role reversal, allowing the student to act as supervisor and demonstrate components of patient care, observe performance and offer constructive feedback.

b) Students should apply factual material to practical problems rather than just accumulating facts.

Teachers can help them to do this by using a problem-based approach. Start with

113

practical problems in the clinic or ward and encourage students to analyse the problems and use their knowledge to work out possible solutions or management of the problems. Patient-centred discussions, routine ward rounds or office hand-over conferences can be organised with this aim in mind.

c)   Students should be carefully supervised.

They should receive adequate feedback on their developing skills and have opportunities for progressive improvement.

d)   Supervisors should be supportive.

Supervisors should be sensitive to the fact that students may be uncomfortable in dealing with patients or the community until they become more confident of their abilities. Clinical supervisors or teachers should avoid harsh criticism and help students to develop confidence by encouraging students to discuss their reactions to their new roles. Fishel and Johnson (1981) have described a three-way conference between student, supervisor and educator which is intended to encourage students to explore their own needs and potential and to prevent the potential problems which arise in the triangular situation in which three parties are involved but only two of the three meet on any given occasion for different purposes. Such a situation frequently gives rise to misunderstanding, discontinuity and loss of accountability with a resultant suboptimal learning environment for the student.

e)   Supervisors should be aware of and comfortable in a variety of roles which make up the supervisor's task.

Activity:
List the main components of the clinical
supervisor's task as you know it.

Feedback:
　　An excellent analysis of the supervisor's
roles has been done for teacher education (Turney
et al, 1983). The roles can also be applied to the
nursing supervisor. In brief they can be summarised
as:

i) Manager:　　　This role includes the success-
　　　　　　　　　ful planning and organising of
　　　　　　　　　the practicum, and the develop-
　　　　　　　　　ment of common understanding,
　　　　　　　　　cooperation and morale of all
　　　　　　　　　participants. This role builds
　　　　　　　　　the setting which facilitates
　　　　　　　　　the pursuit of all the other
　　　　　　　　　roles.

ii) Counsellor:　This role is based on
　　　　　　　　　sensitivity and concern for the
　　　　　　　　　student as a person and as a
　　　　　　　　　developing nurse. It helps the
　　　　　　　　　student develop positive
　　　　　　　　　attitudes, resolve concerns,
　　　　　　　　　clarify behaviours and cooperate
　　　　　　　　　with others.

iii) Instructor:　This role includes skills such
　　　　　　　　　as demonstrating, presenting
　　　　　　　　　ideas, questioning and guiding
　　　　　　　　　problem - solving in special
　　　　　　　　　tutorials and conferences.

iv) Observer:　　The observer role is concerned
　　　　　　　　　with systematically viewing and
　　　　　　　　　recording accurate data on the
　　　　　　　　　performance of the student in
　　　　　　　　　the clinical setting.

v) Feedback:　　Through this role the supervisor
　　　　　　　　　conveys to the student nurse
　　　　　　　　　selected information arising
　　　　　　　　　from the observation of
　　　　　　　　　performance. The main purpose of
　　　　　　　　　this feedback is to assist the
　　　　　　　　　student to gauge progress and
　　　　　　　　　plan ways of surmounting
　　　　　　　　　difficulties.

vi) Evaluator: The evaluator role is concerned
                     with making sound judgements
                     about the level of the student's
                     development as a nurse in rela-
                     tion to the aims of the clinical
                     experience. The evaluator role,
                     if not sensitively and support-
                     ively played could potentially
                     conflict with the counsellor
                     role since the making of
                     judgements about the student
                     almost inevitably poses a threat
                     to the student.

(From Turney et al. 1983, p. 4).

   Awareness of these components of the
supervisor's role assists nurse educators and
supervisors to analyse their relationships with
students and to discover whether there are
deficiencies or imbalances which might be corrected
in order to provide an optimal clinical learning
experience.
   We have covered quite a number of important
points in planning and carrying out effective
clinical learning experiences. The next activity
asks you to reflect on what we have covered and to
integrate it into a plan that you would be able to
use in your own particular situation.

Activity:
Make a checklist which you can use to help you
in planning clinical training for students
that you teach.

Feedback:
     Clinical training should involve **learning by
doing.** It is difficult but valuable experience
which should not be wasted on teaching which could
take place just as well in the classroom. Adequate
preparation of students, supervisors and the other
people who are part of the clinical setting is
essential if learning by doing is to occur in the
clinical placement. Given this sine qua non for
clinical teaching and learning the following points

may be helpful reminders when planning clinical placements for your students.

1. Define goals for clinical work
    Have you decided whether you want your students to:
    a) learn skills and procedures?
    b) deal with real problems?
    c) understand the realities of the nurse's job?
    d) develop attitudes?
        or achieve all of these objectives?

    Remember each clinical experience must be accompanied by a clear statement about what students are expected to achieve during that experience.

2. Plan clinical work
    Are you going to involve the clinical staff and supervisors in planning objectives and methods?
    What experiences will you provide in the classroom to prepare students for the real situation when they enter the clinical placement?
    Will clinical staff and supervisors be trained in effective supervision?

3. Implement clinical work
    Will you:
    a) involve patients and/or community groups in the teaching?
    b) ensure that students' roles and tasks are explicit and understood?
    c) encourage students to perform real tasks and use their own judgement?
    d) use a problem-based approach which allows students to discover appropriate strategies or plan interventions?
    e) provide adequate supervision and feedback on performance?
    f) encourage students to take responsibility for their own learning?
    g) devise ways to assess student performance 'on-the-job' and to provide progressive feedback as an integral part of learning?

    Methods of assessing clinical performance are discussed in Chapter 7.

    We have said that clinical learning offers the

students opportunities to become involved in planning and undertaking their own education. The next section of this chapter deals specifically with methods to help students become independent learners.

INDEPENDENT LEARNING

Independent learning is a term which creates a lot of confusion. Perhaps the easiest way to define it is:

Independent learning is a process in which learners are encouraged to take increasing personal responsibility for achieving learning objectives through their own efforts and at their own pace.

Some examples of independent learning are:

- self-instructional learning units
- continuing education through reading
- elective subjects within training courses
- correspondence courses.

Independence of the learner varies according to who makes the decisions about what to learn and how to learn it.

Total independence of the learner occurs when the learner decides on the objectives of the learning, the methods for learning and the criteria for assessment, in other words when learning is self-directed. Total dependence of the learner occurs when the teacher decides on the objectives, methods and criteria for assessment, in other words when learning is teacher-directed.

A continuum of learning which ranges from totally student-directed to totally teacher directed can be described in the following way.

Student-directed learning

Student decides objectives, methods and assessment.

Student decides objectives and methods. Teacher decides assessment in consultation with student.

Increasing
independence ⇧

Student and teacher discuss and negotiate on objectives methods and assessment

Teacher decides objectives. Student chooses methods. Teacher decides criteria for assessment.

Teacher decides objectives and assessment and recommends a variety of methods.

Teacher decides objectives, methods and assessments.

Teacher-directed learning

Very few professional training courses are totally self-directed. However, there are advantages in encouraging students to be more self-directed in their learning.

The advantages are:
1. If learners set themselves problems to solve or tasks to perform they are more motivated by curiosity or interest to learn the relevant information and to remember it. Teachers can contribute by providing guidance on the scope of problems which can realistically be tackled within specific time periods.
2. Self-directed learners learn how to learn as well as just learning facts. New facts continually replace the old facts learned in training and nurses may quickly become out of

date unless they know how to discover and learn new facts as they become available. Continuing education depends heavily on the nurses' ability to recognise what he or she needs to learn and to seek opportunities for learning it formally or informally.

3. Self-directed learners become more experienced in working without close supervision so that when they enter their jobs as nurses they are more confident of their own abilities and do not have to rely on someone else to tell them what to do. If they have had experience in self-assessment and self-determination of what they need to know they will recognise their own limitations and know how to overcome them.

4. Self-directed learners come to realise that the classroom or training school is not the only place where learning occurs. Many important sources of knowledge and skills learning exist in everyday activities in the home and community. Self-directed learners are encouraged to use these resources instead of relying on information provided only by the teachers. Knowing how to use these resources will be an important part of the nurse's job.

Learning in nursing schools is largely teacher-directed whereas most learning that nurses experience <u>after</u> they have finished training must be self-directed.

Nursing training should prepare students to be self-directed so that they can take responsibility for their own continuing education when they are working in the community or hospital.

Activity:
Write down as many ways as you can think of to help <u>your</u> students to become self-directed or independent learners.

Feedback:
Introducing the idea of independent learning

to students is not always easy. Some may have experienced a degree of self-directed learning in their previous secondary or tertiary education and may be familiar with it and able to benefit from it from the beginning. Many students, however, are not confident enough to take responsibility for their own learning. They expect the teacher to tell them what to learn, how to learn it and whether they have learned it well. It may be wise to introduce independent learning experiences gradually. This allows both you and your students to become familiar with the particular demands and responsibilities of the new roles that you are required to play. Coombe and her coworkers (1981) have described a workshop which gradually introduces nurses to concepts of self-directed learning. Some other specific approaches that you might like to try are listed below:

1.   Offer students a choice of topic.
      Of course there are some things in nursing that students must all know or be able to do and you must help students to master those 'must know' objectives. However there are also many topics which are enriching, which contribute to the nurse's ability to do the job but which are not essential for it. No student will ever be able to learn all there is to know about nursing and so, once the essential knowledge and skills have been mastered students can be offered a choice of topics which particularly interest them. Most schools offer elective terms or programs in their curricula, however electives can also be offered within specific subjects. For example students might undertake a special reading assignment relevant to a patient for whom they have been given responsibility, or they may be given the opportunity to participate in and report on a community aid project.
      Your student would of course need to discuss the aims, scope, resources and criteria for assessment of the independent project with you before starting, but within certain guidelines could be encouraged to develop the study as independently as possible.
2.   Vary the scope and depth of topics to be covered.
      Basic material can be taught in class and more

121

advanced material can be provided in libraries or resource centres to allow students to follow up material in which they have a greater interest. Students could be encouraged to go beyond class work and to further their skills or knowledge by spending free time engaged in extra reading or activities with you or a group of other interested students. Incentives for this extra work could take the form of opportunity to earn extra credits towards the course assessment. Swanson and Dalsing (1980) have described the use of independent study in this way as a curriculum expander.

3.   Provide alternative methods for learning.
      Providing a variety of resources and experiences for learning helps students to discover which methods they prefer and which types of activity or resources help them to learn best. For example, some students learn best by reading, some by listening or discussing. If students are given the opportunity to try a variety of methods they will learn more about how to learn effectively in the future.

4.   Provide students with problems to solve.
      Students who are involved actively in learning through solving problems will remember what they have learned better than they would if the same information had been given to them by the teacher. In addition they will have learned an approach to solving problems which will be very useful to them when they are presented with nursing problems in the course of their work.
      As students become more adept at the process of problem-solving they may discover or generate problems for themselves to solve as part of their elective or practicum studies. Problem-solving is an important approach to the development of independent learners because it requires students to proceed through the following steps, seeking answers to their own questions as they go:
            i)   What is the problem - what are the components of the problem?
           ii)   What information or skills will be needed to solve the problem?
          iii)   Where can the information be found?
           iv)   How can the necessary skills be developed?

v) How should the knowledge and skills be applied to solve the problem?
vi) Did the solution work - might there have been a better one?

Since the problem-solving process depends on students identifying, finding and applying needed information and skills the teacher should act only as guide and advisor rather than as giver of information or provider of solutions.

5.   Consider using self-instructional course units.

If self-instructional programs are available they allow students to learn at their own pace and at the time of their choosing whether a teacher is present or not. Students can use these materials to learn basic information so that the time they spend with the teacher can be used to help them overcome special difficulties or to increase their level of skill or understanding. The student becomes more independent because it is his or her responsibility to discuss individual learning needs with the teacher rather than relying on the teacher to prescribe everything that should be learned.

6.   Provide opportunities for self-assessment.
Students should have frequent opportunities to assess their own performance. The ability to set criteria for personal performance and to gauge performance against those criteria is a critical professional skill for the nurse. Initially students may need guidance in setting criteria and in evaluating themselves against those criteria, however if results of self-assessment are checked with the teacher and guidance provided students can learn to improve the accuracy of self-assessments. A useful adjunct to self-directed learning and self-assessment is the contracting system in which the student contracts with the instructor to achieve specific objectives. The objectives and methods for the study are agreed in consultation and the student is encouraged to develop criteria by which his or her achievement of objectives of the study can be judged. Once the criteria have been agreed to by both parties then the student is able to assess his or her own work accurately. This

123

system also allows students to contract for certain grades. Knowles (1975) gave a general description of this method and Kruse and Fagerbarger (1982) have described its application in nursing education.

7.   Get to know your students.
     If you know your students as individuals and if you demonstrate interest and concern for their needs and their professional development, students will feel more able to take risks, to reveal their uncertainties and their difficulties, in the confidence that you are there to help rather than to judge. Development of self-confidence in learning which leads to the ability to be a self-directed professional depends on the students' preparedness to take these risks. This is particularly true in the area of clinical learning which is a source of anxiety for most students and many teachers.

Activity:
You will have recognized by now that the teacher's tasks in self-directed or independent learning are quite different from the teacher's tasks in traditional teacher-directed learning.

Complete the table overleaf which contrasts the two sets of tasks in each of the areas of educational planning.

	Teacher's tasks in teacher-directed learning	Teacher's tasks in student-directed learning
Objectives		
Content		
Methods		
Feedback		
Assessment		

Feedback:

Teacher's tasks in teacher-directed learning	Teacher's tasks in student-directed learning
Define learning objectives.	Help students to define appropriate learning objectives or problems to investigate.
Provide information in lectures, handouts, books.	Act as a resource to guide students seeking information which will help them achieve their objectives.
Design teaching methods and resources to help students learn.	Make resources available and act as a guide to available facilities which students might seek.
Provide feedback on performance.	Encourage students to provide their own feedback before submitting work to the teacher for assessment
Assess students' achievements of learning objectives.	Work with students to achieve a mutual assessment of the strengths and weaknesses of their independent study project.

The teacher's role in student-directed learning is mainly as a guide, a helper, and a source of encouragement to strengthen the students' own efforts and abilities. As students become more independent they will have less need for guidance, help and encouragement and will be able to find their own way to suitable resources and provide quite accurate judgements of the quality of their own work. That is the ultimate goal of independent learning.

If all of this is beginning to worry you because it seems too different from your usual practice or because you doubt your students' ability, be encouraged by three things:

1. **Independent learning should not be isolated learning.** Students will always need opportunities to interact with their teachers and with each other. Learning how to participate in a group and how to give and receive support and feedback are essential for the development of independent learning skills.

2. **Independent learning** is an important skill for nurses to develop but it is **only one of many skills** they must have. You should provide some opportunities for students to develop it but you need not do all of your teaching that way. A variety of teaching and learning methods is essential. Too much independent learning can be just as frustrating or boring as too many lectures.

3. **Independent learning does not require something extra** or special from your students. What it requires is that they learn to use experience and skills which they already possess.

When students attend a nursing school they know they have much to learn and they feel that the teachers have all of the answers to their questions. They tend to disregard their own knowledge as irrelevant or unimportant in comparison with that of the teacher. You as the teacher must try to help them recognise the importance of what they can contribute to their own and other students' learning.

SUMMARY

This chapter has covered a variety of teaching and learning methods each of which is suited to different educational needs. Of course there is some overlap between methods and what they can achieve. You should aim to use a variety of methods to give your students practice in working in a variety of ways, and you should, if your facilities permit, use those methods best suited to your learning objectives and to your personal talents and preferences.

To summarise the main points we have covered in this unit, try the next Activity.

Activity:
Make a list of the main educational purposes for using <u>each</u> of the following teaching/learning methods:

    Lectures
    Small group tutorials
    Role play
    Supervised clinical and field work
    Demonstrations
    Independent learning.

Feedback:
Each of these methods has special capabilities which make it more useful for some types of learning than others. You, the teacher must choose which methods you prefer to use in your class. While some methods may be best suited to some objectives they may be unsuitable for other reasons which are unique to your situation. For this reason it is not possible to lay down absolute rules which will help you to decide. The following should be used only as a guide.

Use lectures if you want to:
- provide a structure to guide students in learning a topic
- give an overview of a complex topic
- provide perspective and emphasise parts of the topic

- provide information which is not available elsewhere.

Supplement the lecture with handouts, discussions and audio-visual aids when appropriate.

Use small group tutorials if you want to:
- involve students as active participants
- develop skills in teamwork and cooperation
- develop manual or communication skills
- provide practice in applying knowledge to problems or tasks
- promote new ideas and attitudes
- allow for clarifying understanding of a topic.

Use role play activities if you want to:
- explore emotions involved with a topic
- try new behaviour and attitudes in a safe setting similar to the real one
- explore relationships and why people behave as they do.

Use clinical or field work if you want to:
- teach practical skills and procedures
- provide real life practice in dealing with patients' problems
- provide self-awareness of on-the-job capabilities
- expose students to suitable role models.

Use demonstrations if you want to:
- provide visual experience of events or procedures which are difficult to describe
- give an overview of a task or procedure before students begin to practise
- set a problem for students to solve.

Use independent learning if you want to:
- help students learn how to rely on their own judgement
- help students become increasingly independent
- encourage students to learn outside the classroom
- prepare students for lifelong continuing education.

129

CHAPTER 5

CONTEMPORARY PRACTICES IN TEACHING AND LEARNING

Humanising health care has become a priority
for nurses just as it has for most health workers.
Technology and technological change have the power
to both elevate and degrade the care that nurses
give. Teachers of nurses are therefore in a
position of paramount importance in assisting
students to work their way through the ethical,
moral and value conflicts that will confront them
from time to time.

We have selected values, human rights and
ethical dilemmas for attention in this chapter as
these aspects of contemporary nursing are gaining
in importance as ethical problems increase.
Teachers themselves are sometimes faced with
ethical dilemmas in teaching and in nursing
practice. They must also give support to students
and colleagues who may be seeking to resolve an
ethical dilemma.

**By the end of this chapter you should have examined
some of the issues in teaching ethics and you
should be able to design and manage learning
sessions for students to increase their skills in:**
> **clarifying values**
> **discerning human rights**
> **analysing ethical dilemmas.**

While the methods described in the previous
chapter are appropriate for teaching most subjects
and are appropriate in most situations, some
adaptations are suggested in this chapter. The
alternatives are offered to complement your usual
teaching methods and to add to your repertoire of
teaching skills. It is for you to decide whether
they are appropriate for your purposes in assisting
students in your particular program.

130

Curriculum issues

At the outset it should be said that to be most effective, teaching about values, human rights, moral reasoning and ethical decision-making should be an integral part of the curriculum. This is not to say that a large proportion of curriculum time should be devoted to those areas, but rather to make the point that adding-on to an established curriculum is less than satisfactory and leads to teaching that is fragmented and often not in tune with the philosophical base of the program. On the other hand a curriculum that has been designed from concepts such as the nature of humankind or human needs, would have identified the salient issues of values and human rights, and would have included the need for ethical decision-making as a required skill.

Rather than a substantial content area we are dealing with a process - a way of thinking - and the personal development that accompanies it. When such a process is embedded in the curriculum students and teachers are enabled to progress from a beginning understanding of values to a mature skill, by the end of the program.

However, in spite of the pitfalls many teachers would prefer to design a few brief sessions than none at all because of the need to include this important dimension in nursing practice and education.

Teaching and Learning Issues

What is taught in nursing sometimes has little to do with what students want to know. Deciding what to teach (Chapter 2) and arranging the conditions most likely to bring about learning (Chapter 3) have their foundation in accepted educational principles, so also does the design of teaching sessions (Chapter 4). Yet, in spite of the expertise a teacher may possess in modifying educational principles for a particular learning situation, and the enthusiasm brought to the teaching of a subject, students often respond more to the pressures for socialisation into the mores of hospital practice than to life-long learning skills of gaining knowledge and applying it to practice.

It is, of course, not surprising that the hidden curriculum (socialisation process) makes students want to know how to master skills, behaviours and attitudes which will bring rewards of approval and acceptance within a hierarchical system. Personal growth is often questionably attributed to the molding and shaping process of socialisation. On the other hand, the pressures on teachers to teach a packed course and to cover the content, sometimes results in the selection of teaching materials and experiences that are often routine, dull and yawningly boring.

Materials that are repeated many times lose their capacity to inspire, to spark imagination or to encourage spontaneity. The important links between what is being taught and the student's personal growth are tenuous, if ever made explicit, and the rewards for students are virtually non-existent. Most students want to know more than what to do, or what to know; they are, 'whole' people too, and they search for meaning. What does this mean for me? How ought I to behave? What is 'right' action for me in this or that situation?

The teaching of values, human rights and ethical decision-making is as vulnerable (or more so) to the powers of the hidden curriculum as any other area in the curriculum. It may be more vulnerable because the students' questions are ethical questions and are not answered effectively by current socialisation pressures. Some nurses believe that until professional socialisation is linked with skills such as decision-making, use of self, ethical understanding, curiosity, commitment and caring, and until approval is shown for these attainments, the search for meaning in nursing will be limited.

Certainly, the standards of practice developed by professional associations point to levels of expertise and high standards of care to which nurses should aspire and on such a professional plane we could say that the search for the meaning of nursing's service to the community has begun. For individual students, however, the search for meaning is personal, holds the key to personal growth and has the potential for lifting ideas out of the everyday commonplace to increasing levels of understanding of themselves and others. It is this dimension which is so important to capture in teaching values, human rights and ethics. The rigidity and blandness suggested by formal codes of ethics should in no way prejudice us about the nature of thinking about ethical issues.

Issues of practice

Professional nursing practice which fosters creativity, imagination and curiosity, and is open-ended can be observed in many areas of practice: the hospice movement; neighbourhood teaching centres; specially designed children's clinics (Johnston, 1979); and remote areas nursing, to name but a few. The search for meaning in professional practice is also evident in 'curious nurse clinicians'. Reading Norris's (1975) article "Restlessness: A nursing phenomenon in search of meaning" is to be swept up in the excitement of discovering the extraordinary from what nurses see every day. To engage in reflective thinking about what has been observed, is another dimension of ethical analysis.

Summary

In summary then, to be effective, a course in ethics (including values and human rights) is, preferably:

- **integrated within the curriculum**
- **designed to facilitate the personal growth of students**
- **provides time and guidance for reflective and critical thinking**
- **produces skills to use in the resolution of ethical dilemmas of real people.**

VALUES - CLARIFICATION

Since there are many definitions of value, we will quote one - 'those elements that show how a person has decided to use his life' - (Raths et al. 1966) and suggest that you will find slight variations in Simon (1972), Uustal, (1977) and Reilly (1978).

Activity:
You have offered to take responsibility for the introduction of a series of sessions on ethics for students in a basic program. The course has three components: values, human rights and ethics. You are preparing to

teach the values component. What do you hope
your students will derive from it?

Feedback:
You may be teaching in a program where ethics
(including values and human rights) is a separate
course or an elective subject. In that case you
will be able to plan a course so that time is
available for students to reflect on some of the
issues in **value development** and **values-clarification.** Your expectation would be that the students
would **gain an understanding of the values they
hold.** This would serve as a preparation for ethical
decision-making later as they take more responsibility in the care of patients. On the other hand
your program may not devote so much time to ethics
but may acknowledge the importance of values by
allotting special sessions during an intensive care
or coronary care course.
There   are   alternative   arrangements   for
including values-clarification in the program
although a whole session may not be given over to
the topic. For example, in clinical practice or
community placements, the pre- and post-clinical
conference can offer a special opportunity for
choosing and clarifying values. For example, the
knowledge necessary for nursing a patient with
multiple fractures and internal injuries following
a car accident could be followed by revision of the
skills of observation, technical treatment, basic
care and planning a rehabilitation program. Lastly,
the fact that the patient has been charged with
drunken driving in the accident which killed a
child, calls into question the effectiveness of
nursing the patient if the values dimension has not
been faced openly and explored.
Values-clarification can also be built into
subject matter. Perhaps this is obvious to most
teachers but it is fairly common in practice to
find that teachers may exhibit their own values on
a particular issue (for example the right to life
movement) but omit values-clarification as a means
of opening up or expanding students' skill in
recognising their own values. Needless to say, the
important point is that at some time during the
course students need to **learn the process of
valuing.**

In summary your learning objectives for students in the values component of the course in ethics would be, broadly:

- gaining an understanding of our own personal values
- using the process of valuing
- recognising personal and professional values

Activity:
You have decided to introduce first year students to values-clarification. As this will be a departure from their usual format of lectures and group discussion on the substantive content of the course, how will you prepare the students for your session?

Feedback:
You could apply the principles of 'advance organisers' discussed in Chapter 3. This would help students to prepare for learning about values by linking it to their past learning or experiences.

For example, questions related to a recent class, such as:

During the lecture in paediatric nursing several students took issue with the case history presented of child abuse. What was your view? Why?

Select an issue that came up in a clinical session recently. Make yourself a button supporting the issue and wear it for a day. What reaction did you get?

Ask five friends, colleagues or family members to complete a sentence or two, such as;

At the moment I _____
In my view health care _____

(The topic of the sentence should be chosen to provide the link with a previous session.)
Bring the completed statements to the values class.

As well as acting as advance organisers, the answers students bring to class provide a warming-up period at the beginning of the session. It is often useful to have a poster wall of issues to work from. Students' contributions written or drawn on butcher's paper can be displayed anonymously at first, then acknowledged later when the group is felt to be supportive for its members.

Activity:
As a facilitator in the values-clarification session you will have chosen an informal setting and arranged a comfortable atmosphere and encouraged the display of posters around the room. What will you do next?

Feedback:
The first time you conduct a values-clarification session you will probably over-prepare for it. That is an advantage as you can use whichever strategy appears to be appropriate to the group's progress. The methods you choose depend on how well you know the group and also on your perception of the importance of the development and clarification of values.

First, it is important for you to explain to the students the purpose and the ground rules of the session: - 'you will learn ways of valuing-not a particular set of values; it is for you to discover where you stand on issues you may be facing; you are allowed to have 'time out' on an issue if you don't wish to discuss your particular stance.'

Second, you may also consider it is important to spend a short few minutes confiding your understanding of the process of valuing to the group. For instance, you may wish the group to be aware that you recognise in teachers, parents and authorities several forms of valuing, for example:

Moralising   - pressing on others one's view
                   of what is right or wrong.
Laissez faire -   leaving values up to chance.
Modelling   - trying to make practice and
                   ideals match
Values-clarification - building one's own
                       value system
                       (Simon, 1978)

The group's reaction would be very interesting at this point and could be elicited by asking students to write a slogan to fit each of the four types, then discussing the comparative forms of valuing. For example:

VALUE FORM		SLOGAN
Moralising	-	people who don't care don't deserve care.
Laissez faire	-	who cares?
Modelling	-	I care, between 9 am and 5 pm
Values clarification	-	caring costs, but I choose to care.

Third, with the group relaxed and the butcher's paper wall posters as a back drop, the theoretical framework of values-clarification would be introduced, preferably as a brief handout with discussion. The purpose would be to use the theory for guidance in clarifying the values brought to class.

Raths' Theory of Valuing (1966)

The human being can arrive at values by an intelligent process of choosing, prizing and behaving.

Choosing	-	1	Freely
		2	From alternatives
		3	After thoughtful consideration of the consequences of each alternative
Prizing	-	4	Cherishing, being happy with choice
		5	Willing to affirm the choice publicly
Acting	-	6	Doing something with the choice
		7	Repeatedly, in some pattern of life.

Fourth, returning to the wall posters, group members could explain the value they had identified, obtain clarification and consider the consequences of an alternative choice (Steps 1, 2 and 3 above) to test the strength of the value (Step 4 above). A useful strategy is to involve the whole group in forming a continuum. This is done by individuals taking a position on an imaginary line from positive at one end of the line to the negative at the opposite pole. The students place themselves at appropriate points on the continuum to express the strength of their view. This often results in clarification as re-thinking and re-positioning occurs following hearing from other students the justification they have given for their position. The aim is to enable students to obtain feedback on their statement of the values they purport to hold. This strategy is also a dramatic way of demonstrating that issues are rarely clear cut with a black or white decision.

Fifth, being comfortable with the choice of a value leads to a willingness to affirm it publicly. (Step 5 above). In class this can be done by sending an imaginary telegram; an 'I urge you' telegram. Blank telegram forms can be supplied to add a touch of realism and the strategy works best if the subject of the telegram is a topical issue and the recipient is sufficiently prominent to excite imaginative messages. For example, an 'I urge you' telegram to the Minister for Health following the decision to close city hospitals or reduce a community health program could generate a number of values:

I urge you to close hospital X, not my hospital
I urge you to close more beds, this country is oversupplied
I urge you to think of students who need sufficient clinical material to learn on

The telegram should be made public, the sender should give the justification, aided by the group who should question and comment until the value is affirmed or denied.

A criticism of such strategies is that the activity is an end in itself and fails to carry over into the students' learning. For some students this criticism would apply. According to Simon (1978, p. 20) there is empirical evidence that students who have taken part in values-clarification have become less apathetic, less flighty, less conforming as well as less over-dissenting. They are more zestful and energetic, more critical in their thinking and are more likely to follow through on decisions (p. 20).

Another criticism is that the act of choosing a value allows the individual to accept or reject certain values. Purtilo (1983,p. 216) points out that in nursing and the health professions generally, there are some values that logically follow if a concept such as 'treating the whole patient' is accepted. The reasoning is that the 'whole' person is not only a physical, emotional or spiritual being but also a moral being. Values such as quality of life, right of choice, and self-determination are part of a professional ethic which, it is assumed, members of the profession not only accept but practise. Raths' (1966) theory of valuing is composed of seven processes, the last two being concerned with acting on one's belief. The assumption here is that the person will indicate what action will result from possessing and affirming a particular value.

Sixth, this would be an appropriate point to clarify with the group what congruence they can identify between their personal values and the professional values they have observed so far in their experience. Depending on the level of your group you could proceed by:
   (1) setting group tasks based on the students' suggestions of points for clarification
   (2) setting group tasks by assigning to each a clause from the international code of nursing ethics and comparing the values expressed in it with the personal values affirmed earlier by the group.

As a summary, a plan of possible strategies is given below. The size of your student group, the time and the resources available together with your personal preferences and the level of your group will determine which of the strategies you wish to use or adapt.

Summary of Suggested Plan for values-clarification sessions

Objective	Teacher activity	Student activity
	Prepares group by giving advance organisers. Arranges room. Sets tone.	Obtains information. Records on wall posters.
Uses the process of valuing	.Gives ground rules .Gives own examples of valuing .Introduces Raths' theory in stages. .Steps 1,2 & 3	.Discusses ground rules .Writes slogans & discusses values .Discusses theory .Applies steps 1, 2 & 3 of theory to values chosen from those recorded on wall posters
Gains an understanding of personal values	. Step 4 . Step 5	.Affirms and clarifies a value publicly .Acts on the value by an 'I urge' telegram
Recognises personal & professional values	. Step 6 .Sets up group task and facilitates group interaction Summarises .Foreshadows work on human rights. Makes links. Closes session.	.Compares personal and professional values

HUMAN RIGHTS: CONTEMPORARY NURSING ISSUES

We have now reached the point where we move from designing learning strategies for clarifying personal or individual values to those for teaching about shared values, or universal rights. However, there is merit in designing your sessions on human rights so that a direct link is made with the work your students have done on their own values. The reason is that students find the study of human rights (important though it is) to be remote if it drifts too soon into abstract statements and official declarations. After all, the aim of humanising relationships in health care becomes meaningless to students if the method of teaching about human rights is so formal that it is routine, dull and boring, in a word - dehumanising.

> **'What we have to respect are real people, not abstractions or sentimental idealisations.'**
> (Kamenka and Tay, 1981)

The purpose of teaching about human rights in a nursing course is to develop skills in analysing critically the basic human rights that are our concern because of our responsibilities as health professionals.
We should try to be as clear as possible about the learning objectives for students in these sessions. Again, we are assisting them in learning skills, and in shaping attitudes.

Activity:
What are the learning objectives you consider are important for students to achieve by the end of the session(s) on human rights?

Feedback:
Not a little confusion may be generated by the terms 'teaching human rights' or 'teaching about human rights' as if there exists somewhere, a body of knowledge called 'human rights.'

> **'Human rights in themselves are not matters of knowledge in the way that chemistry or biology are matters of knowledge.'** (Singer, 1981).

141

Does your list of learning objectives include the following?

- Developing an awareness of own rights and the rights of others
- raising own consciousness concerning the human rights of groups who need to have their rights defended
- becoming sensitive to human rights as a humanising element in nursing practice
- sharpening critical skills in analysing human rights.

Preparing to teach about human rights

Activity:
Although the aim of your session is to assist students to analyse human rights and to sharpen their critical skills rather than to teach a subject, you will need to have a working knowledge of human rights as well as skills in managing the sessions. How will you prepare for a session on human rights?

Feedback:
1. Get to know what your students know (or don't know). Singer (1981) speaks with some authority as a teacher and writer on human rights. In his view a considerable percentage of the university students he teaches seem unaware of the existence of disadvantaged groups in the community. There is a strong possibility that nursing students are more aware because of their contact with health care but may also have 'blind spots' to other areas of disadvantage in the wider community.
2. Be aware of the role of the ombudsman in your city and have a working knowledge of the human rights problems that your ombudsman deals with.
3. Read about the doctrine of human rights in such general texts as Fenner (1980), Kamenka and Tay (eds) (1981); human rights in health professional education and

practice, Purtilo (1983); human rights and nursing, Benoliel (1983).

4. Remember that your human rights session is primarily a consciousness-raising session to prepare your students for their role in recognising the rights of patients and in assisting patients to understand the implications of those rights.

5. Resist the urge to prepare your session as if it were a mini lecture on human rights. First, you risk the charge of moralising because you will find it hard to avoid advocating a set of values which could be at variance with your students and belongs in the values-clarification sessions.
Second, the aim of the session is for the student to engage in an analysis of human rights and to reflect on or work through the issues involved. This expectation implies that the teacher also works through the issues with the students. This is a clear indication to students that human rights is not a specialised subject to be learned but a way of thinking and behaving. As a role model of an analyser and critical thinker you are enabling the student to observe and work with a real person.

6. Become skilled in identifying fallacies in analysing human rights arguments. Listen to live debates on radio; attend community meetings on local rights issues; read the report of a skilled analyst. Study the steps in moral reasoning: general (Phenix, 1966; Fenner, (1980) and nursing (Aroskar, 1980; Purtilo, 1983).

Involving your students in human rights issues

Activity:
There are several ways to teach about human rights. How would you design a learning session to involve your students in learning about the rights of real people?

Feedback:

If you have read Andrews and Hutchinson's (1981) article you might have considered using a similar strategy for your session on human rights. Andrews and Hutchinson developed eight stereotyped responses of people to the problem of the exploitation of patients as 'clinical material' for student learning. Each student took a position on the stereotypes and defended it. After the group's discussion and the teacher's prompting, an analysis of each position was achieved. The aim was for students to analyse their comments and to identify the presuppositions which formed the basis of their beliefs. For the teacher, the role taken was one of clarifying the students' views pointing out inconsistencies and leading students towards an understanding of ethical reasoning. An analysis of human rights could be done in much the same way. Typical stereotyping is not hard to find and it is possible that the students themselves could suggest common stereotypes from their own experiences as citizens in the community.

Kamenka and Tay (1981) and other workers in the same volume stress the importance of considering human rights in their context, not as an abstraction in a vacuum. In choosing an universal right for analysis in your session it is important to set it in its context so that students will be able to relate easily to the problem.

Take for example, the topical issue of equal opportunity, set in the context of entry into tertiary education or the right to work. Stereotyped positions on this issue would readily come to the minds of students as many of their peers are probably affected. For example, such assertions as the following are frequently heard:

> married women in the work force reduce the
> availability of jobs
> the job market favours 'types' of
> applicants
> employers don't care
> the government should do more
> people prefer handouts
> ... and so on.

A similar approach has been used by Carlson (1970) but instead of individual students taking a position, two groups prepare to face each other with prepared arguments for dealing with a series of human rights problems. The strategy resembles a debate but the teacher's role is not as an adjudicator but a clarifyer of views, facilitator of critical analysis and supporter of students caught in the cross-fire of contentious debate.

Human rights and nursing practice

As your students gain skill in analysing human rights issues and depending on their level of maturity and their experience in nursing and health care, you and your students will want to move the sessions more into the realm of nursing practice. There is value in beginning with issues outside the field of nursing rather than moving immediately into nursing issues with junior students who lack sufficient experience and whose relationships with patients needs to grow 'naturally' person to person in the beginning stages of their learning to nurse. So many pressures: unfamiliarity, and inexperience; stress resulting from the severity of illness or death of patients; emergencies and crises, fill a new student's experience and require time to work through. The added pressure of having students learn to analyse human rights problems at too early a stage is an unwise teaching strategy.

On the other hand, extending the human rights concept from community issues, student issues and finally to patient's rights through a series of experiential strategies has the effect of drawing on the students' personal knowledge and individual values and expanding their understanding to an appreciation of shared values of peers, societal values and eventually to professional values and ethics.

Nursing roles and human rights

Activity:
What roles in nursing or nurse education would you consider important to examine in terms of their opportunity for recognising and defending human rights in health care and education?

Feedback:
    It would be hard to omit any direct contact
role of nurse and patient, or teacher and student
as the basic principle is that human rights are
fundamental   to   harmonious   relationships.   The
dehumanising   potential   of   technological   and
bureaucratic routines are a threat to all of the
participants. Nevertheless there are some roles
specially selected by nurses because of their
heightened awareness of human rights issues or
because their previous training and experience
singles those nurses out as particularly suited to
acting in such a role. For our purposes it is
useful to analyse the role and to involve students
in realising its implications. For example, some of
these roles are:

  • patient advocate
  • change agent
  • academic counsellor
  • consumer activist
  • student-union officer
  • community liaison developer.

Activity:
You have decided to involve your   senior
students in a session aimed at
1) examining the human rights aspects of
   these roles
2) analysing the issues involved for
   patients, nurses, students and teachers.
   How would you structure the session so
   that your aims were reached?

Feedback:
    If you are a confident discussion leader you
could choose to guide the students through a free
ranging discussion. The issues certainly lend
themselves to fruitful discussion and the guides to
managing small groups in the previous chapter will
assist you to draw the group's discussion to
conclusions: However, constraints of time and class
size often demand a structure which allows maximum
opportunity for each student to be involved. A
suggested structuring you could try for a 2 hour
session is:

After a brief introduction to the session
(5-10 minutes)
(1) Distribute the roles of patient-advocate,
change agent and so on, so that each small
group (or individual students or pairs if
your group is very small) is assigned a
role
(2) Provide a brief human rights problem on,
for example,
informed consent
access to information
right of choice
freedom from discrimination
freedom from harassment
self-determination,
and introduce the task. (5 minutes)
(3) Give each group the task of drawing up
a list of responsibilities of the
incumbent of the role so that the rights
of the persons they were most likely to
serve were protected. (Allow approximately
30 mins.)
(4) Without returning to the large group for
discussion the second task for the group
is to draw up a list of rights for their
respective client, patient or students.
(Allow approximately 30 mins.)
(5) Merge the groups, that is,
patient advocate and change agent
consumer activist and liaison
developer
academic counsellor and student union
officer
to provide comparison of the 'Bills of
Rights' (15 mins.)
(6) Returning to the large group, discuss the
issues involved for students, teachers,
patients and clients through group reports
and a summary of the rights identified by
the groups. (20 mins.)

Human rights in specific situations

A useful strategy to use as a summarising
session is a series of trigger films. Careful
choice of the triggers to exemplify the increasing
complexity of human rights problems and to move
from students' problems to patients' problems is
important. For example, a set of three trigger

147

films (Pashuk, 1983) could be used, such as:

(1) A student asks the teacher for justification of the marking scheme in a recent examination and why his result was 'fail!'

(2) A patient refuses to take medication offered by the nurse.

(3) A patient and a nurse seek clarification of a proposed extensive surgical procedure.

If trigger films are not available the scenes could be acted out in role play but the advantage of trigger films is their capacity to sharpen the involvement of students, and to rivet their attention. Usually the vignette is sufficiently short so that the issue portrayed is left without a suggested outcome. Before each vignette the students are asked:

. to imagine you are the nurse (or student)
. what would you say or do?

and to record their responses following each vignette.

Students' responses are usually immediate and very revealing of the strength of their reactions (sometimes even to their own surprise). What they would say or do in the confidential circumstances of the classroom (before the reaction is thought through for its social approval) gives an indication of underlying beliefs and values. Sharing their responses in a small supportive group can extend students' understanding of the human rights at issue. Also, having the opportunity of coming to grips with their own response and affirming or analysing it, is, in itself a humanising experience.

In summary, the purpose of teaching about human rights is to introduce students to a way of thinking about their responsibilities as individuals, citizens and health professionals in preserving and fostering an acceptable set of behaviours (morals or norms) for living and working peacefully and harmoniously together (Purtilo, 1983).

Purtilo's (1983) article gives a summary of the morals and norms appropriate to the health professions:

Duties: do no harm
             be faithful to contracts

```
                      do all one can for the patient

      Rights:         rights of patients
                      rights of health professionals
                      rights of society

      Responsi-
      bilities:       of health professionals
                      of patients
                      of society

      Justice:        seek a fair distribution of
                          resources
                      compensate for injuries.
```

Adhering to these duties, rights, responsibilities, and conditions of justice constitutes the **moral dimension** of the delivery of health care.

NURSES AND ETHICAL DECISION-MAKING

The purpose of teaching ethical analysis and decision-making is to provide for reflective thinking and through such thinking to identify the guidance necessary in resolving ethical problems. Your students in a course of ethics (preceded by values-clarification and discussions on human rights) will no doubt come to these sessions with an expectation that there will be learning materials to assist their reflective thinking. In an important sense therefore, what has been covered by the previous sections represents preparation for learning the complex skill of ethical analysis and decision-making.

As we saw in the last section of this chapter, adhering to duties, rights, responsibilities and fairness is part of the moral dimension of health care. Purtilo (1983) defines the terms morals and ethics neatly:

'Morals are the content of ethical reflection. Ethics is a discipline designed to sort out conflicts among duties, rights or responsibilities. Therefore, ethics analyses problems involving morals'

Explaining the basis of ethical analysis Purtilo continues:

> **'It is useful to think of the moral norms described above (duties, rights, responsibilities, justice) as 'elements' of ethical analysis. These elements can be observed, weighed, assessed and compared when they conflict.'**

Although sometimes in critical situations there is not opportunity for reflective thinking or for weighing all the elements but rather an immediate action is required (for example triage) yet preparation for exercising such a responsibility lies in a careful consideration of the steps involved during a well planned learning session.

> **'The realm of ethics then, is right action, The central concept in this domain is obligation or what ought to be done. The 'ought' here is not an individual but a universal principle of right.'** (Phenix, 1966)

So when a health worker asks - what ought I to do in this situation? - the question calls on more than a clarification of values and human rights but in addition, draws on ethical principles and theories in order to reach a resolution. Obviously, the skill involved is complex and although there are 'tools' to use, it seems preferable to continue an emphasis on the 'way of thinking!' Use of a tool implies some control or power over an object or a situation. What we are implying is really the opposite of a technology; it is the use of imagination, concern, compassion and intellect in the application of a universal principle in order to arrive at a moral solution which will be in the best interests of the person(s) involved.

Activity:
What do you want your students to achieve by the end of your sessions in ethical decision-making?

Feedback:
   First, competence in analysing an ethical problem. Second, skills in applying the steps in ethical decision-making to resolve an ethical dilemma.

1. Competence in analysing an ethical problem. An ethical problem may arise out of everyday situations such as keeping a promise, honoring a contract to produce an outcome; completing a treatment or an assignment or explaining the concept of informed consent so that satisfaction that the patient has understood, has been achieved before the document is signed.

   Some ethical problems border on legal problems. Examples are failing to honour an agreement about the care of a patient and thereby incurring negligence. Legal decisions are therefore called for. However, ethical problems are not dispensed with by a legal decision when an analysis of the situation reveals that an ethical dilemma exists.

A series of questions has been devised to analyse an ethical problem, (Hynes, 1980, p. 20) which, in brief, are:
   (1) What is the medical problem and the corresponding ethical question?
   (2) Who is involved?
   (3) What is the role of each individual involved?
   (4) Am I the decision-maker for either the clinical problem or the ethical issue?
   (5) Having reviewed alternative courses of action, what are the implications of any decision for myself, and those identified in Question 2?
   (6) Does this decision reinforce my general value orientation?

2. Skills in applying the steps in ethical decision-making to resolve an ethical dilemma.

151

Ethical dilemmas are the most perplexing of ethical problems as they involve inter-relationships in which there are conflicts and tensions. Bioethical dilemmas arise in health care when a choice has to be made between two equally unattractive alter-natives. Purtilo (1983) warns that the health professional involved should make certain that it is an ethical dilemma before acting to resolve the situation, as the implications for the patient and the health professional of hasty decisions,are grave.

A four step process of analysis is advocated: (Purtilo, 1983)
'The health professional must ask:
(1) Do I have all the relevant data I can get about this situation?
(2) What kind of moral problem is this?
(3) What are my alternatives for responding?
(4) In the end, what can and should I do to alleviate or attenuate the distress caused by the problem.'

The rise in complexity and frequency of ethical dilemmas in health care has seen the growth of bioethics as a discipline applying ethical thinking to the health sciences (Aroskar, 1980). Choices and conflicts have arisen in issues such as prolongation of human life through the advent of life support systems, increased knowledge of genetics and genetic engineering, increased sophistication in clinical research, in vitro fertilisation and judgement about human life.

The steps in resolving ethical dilemmas have been variously described by Curtin (1978) and Aroskar (1980). Curtin's model includes the factors of background information, identification of ethical components and ethical agents, identification of options, application of principles and resolution.

Aroskar's model for analysing an ethical dilemma consists of three elements: data base, decision theory dimensions, and ethical theories and positions. The analysis of an ethical problem is traced by Aroskar in 'Anatomy of an Ethical Dilemma' (1980) showing how each step in the model is applied.

The difference offered by Curtin (1978) and Aroskar (1980) from the steps advocated by Hynes (1980) and Purtilo (1983) is the addition of the application of ethical theories in order to resolve the dilemma.

In structuring learning sessions so that your students achieve these objectives you could (if time permits) develop separate sessions for each objective.

Activity:
In achieving competence in analysing an ethical problem what skills would you expect of your students?

Feedback:
By this stage having proceeded from values-clarification and human rights considerations, you would be looking for indications that your students could
(1) identify the difference between value judgements and judgements based on evidence
(2) recognise and state their own biases
(3) question critically the basis on which historical decisions in ethical problems have been made
(4) read scholarly articles on bioethics and professional ethics and discuss the issues involved
(5) scrutinise the moral or ethical implications of the ethical position taken in the readings
(6) apply their own insights in the analysis of ethical problems

---

Activity:
In applying the steps of ethical decision-making to resolve an ethical dilemma what skills would you expect of your students by the end of your sessions?

153

Feedback:
Resolving a bioethical dilemma is rarely the responsibility of an individual health professional. The interdisciplinary nature of bioethical issues means that the nurse needs to understand the issues from a number of perspectives and to use the various perspectives in the analysis of ethical issues.

In addition to skills listed above, (1-6) you would probably expect the following:
  (7) develop an adequate framework for decision making
  (8) recognise through studying ethical decisions the practical consequences of the theoretical convictions they hold
  (9) recognise the conflicting rights in particular ethical dilemmas
  (10) debate the need for a systematic ethical analysis in bioethical dilemmas
  (11) discern the role of creative imagination in providing alternatives before a decision is made in resolving an ethical dilemma
  (12) appreciate that ethical decisions demand a maturity able to accept the ambiguity, implications and consequences of decisions. (Mitchell, 1981).

Activity:
What learning sessions will you prepare to enable your students to achieve the objectives and to become competent in the skills listed above?

Feedback:
(1) Mitchell (1981) describes a case study approach he uses in a ethics course. The skills above numbers 7-12 have been adapted from his report of the classes he conducts. He gives a sensitive account of the overview of the course and his role and also describes students' reaction to a number of cases they studied.
(2) Reilly (1978) has proposed a 'dilemma worksheet' in the light of Kohlberg's (1972) theory of stages of moral development.

(3) Davis and Aroskar (1978) and Davis and Krueger (1980) include resources from which learning materials can be structured.

(4) Aroskar (1980) suggests a format of 'ethical rounds' similar to the case study method where actual or hypothetical situations are analysed for their specific ethical dilemmas. Davis (1979) has also used ethical rounds successfully with intensive care nurses.

> **'Whatever learning strategy is used and regardless of the model of analysis employed, it is important to select issues that are appropriate to the students' understanding.'**
> (Lamb, 1982)

In summary, this chapter has dealt with the need to counteract the dehumanising effects of technology in modern health care by sensitising students to the values and human rights that affect daily decisions about the well being of patients and families. The chapter also indicated the importance of including ethics in a nursing curriculum because of the fundamental (but complex) skill of ethical decision-making in which nurses and other health professions are involved to an increasing extent.

No doubt, as you have progressed through this chapter (which deals with the way values, human rights and ethics might be taught), you have questioned many of the assumptions on which the teaching methods are based. If that is so, the chapter will have worked in the way intended. There are often no clear right or wrong prescriptions to follow in teaching this area of nursing practice. Clearly what works with one group may prove unsuccessful with another.

Teachers often find it helpful to pool their unsuccessful attempts at teaching as well as their achievements, so that they can draw upon their experiences in a productive way. This chapter is also a way of facing the values we as teachers hold in our commitment to seeking the most fruitful ways of assisting students to learn to nurse as independent individuals.

Activity:
After progressing through this chapter what
advantages do you see for students in a course
of values-clarification, human rights and
ethics? What challenges for the teacher have
come to mind?

Values-clarification

Challenges for the teacher

- could suggest that students are free to
  choose any set of values in health care
  regardless of professional ethics
- the method of values-clarification may be
  treated superficially
- time-consuming to teach
- demanding of teaching skills.

Benefits for the student

- provides students with a sense of
  assessing their own values and the values
  of others
- leads to values as a principle of action
- enables students to identify their reasons
  for preferring and prescribing one view
  over another
- sensitises students to thinking about
  human rights and professional ethics
- emphasises the valuing aspects of making
  judgements.

Human Rights

Challenges for the teacher

- demanding of intellectual discipline
- demanding of skills in examining issues of
  human rights and facilitating students'
  skills of critical thinking
- leads to examination of the issue of
  students' and teachers' rights

.   could trap teachers into moralising
.   often difficult to shift the emphasis for students from personal values to universal values
.   could make teachers vulnerable to criticism because of lack of substantive content in the area of human rights
.   difficult to retain a focus on students' progress in critical thinking rather than a mastery of content as demanded by other areas of the curriculum.

Benefits for the student

.   draws on values-clarification to explore the value conflicts in health care
.   sensitises students to the rights of disadvantaged groups
.   raises issues of responsibility of nurses to protect the rights of others and of themselves
.   identifies the role of nurses in assisting patients and families to clarify their values, beliefs and rights
.   enables students to examine the concept of rights and obligations
.   assists students to clarify the different kinds of rights
.   prepares students for inter-professional discussion of patient rights in health care.

Ethics

Challenges for the teacher

.   presents a challenge to differentiate between the strategies of nursing process (problem-solving) and ethical decision-making (resolving an ethical dilemma)
.   could make teachers vulnerable to the charge of intellectualising in place of experiencing ethical decision-making in the real situation
.   the ambiguous nature of ethical decisions could create insecurity
.   constant support of students is needed as ethical theories and strategies can only

serve as a guide to resolving a dilemma;
each situation requires personal inputs of
of intuition, experience, maturity and
understanding
. support is also needed for students as
they face the fact that rarely can a
satisfactory resolution to an ethical
dilemma be obtained. Choosing between two
equally unattractive alternatives ensures
that the final conclusion is less than
desirable.

Benefits for the student

. encourages critical thinking as a skill
. legitimises time spent in reflective
thinking
. extends the students' awareness of both
the benefits of high technology and the
drawbacks for individuals caught in
dilemmas of accepting or rejecting the
benefits
. learning the ethical component of nursing
practice is pervasive and contributes to
the students' personal knowledge and
growth
. integrates ethical decision-making into
day-to-day nursing skills
. leads to an open forum between health
professionals.

* * * * * * *

"To be a nurse" Levine (1977) asserts "requires
the willing assumption of ethical responsibility in
every dimension of practice. The nurse enters a
partnership of human experience where sharing
moments in time - some trivial and some dramatic -
leaves its mark forever on each participant. The
willingness to enter with a patient that predica-
ment which he cannot face alone, is an expression
of moral responsibility; the quality of the moral
commitment is a measure of the nurse's excellence."

Chapter 6.

USING LEARNING RESOURCES

The previous chapters in this book have helped you to decide what your students need to know, and to identify some of the types of learning experiences and methods which will be most effective in helping students to learn. This chapter looks in more detail at some of the resources you might use to assist your teaching.

When you have finished this chapter you should be able to assess the resources available to you and choose those which are most appropriate to the learning objectives you have identified. You should also be able to develop some of those resources yourself.

The resources that will be dealt with in this chapter are those which are most commonly used in nursing education. Those resources are people, facilities, handouts, 35mm slides, overhead projection transparencies, videotape and simulations of various types. One important point deserves mention before we start and that is that learning resources need not be very expensive or very sophisticated. For some purposes, simple home-made resources may be more effective than expensive commercially produced materials which are not designed specifically for the needs of your students. For our purposes then resources are any people, facilities, or materials which you can call on to assist you in carrying out your teaching plan.

PEOPLE AS RESOURCES

Activity:
Think of the ways in which you use other people as resources in your teaching. Are there any other possibilities that you would like to try?

Feedback:
Probably the first people you thought of were other tutors or teachers and patients. However, have you thought of using the students themselves as resources? Students can be used as models of living anatomy, they can practise simple procedures on each other, they can play roles to give each other practice in interpersonal relationships and they can also be trained to provide valuable feedback to each other. Most nursing teachers will be familiar with students developing their skills by practising on each other but may not be familiar with the idea that students can learn to assess each other's performance and provide constructive feedback. In situations where there may be a shortage of teachers students should be encouraged to help each other in this way and to become comfortable with giving feedback as well as receiving it from a peer. Peer evaluation is an important professional skill which should be developed from the earliest stages of training.

A more sophisticated use of people as resources in medical education is described by Barrows (1971) who has for many years used 'programmed patients', well individuals who have been trained to simulate certain clinical symptoms and signs.

Be careful that you don't overlook any other resources such as personnel of hospital departments who might welcome the opportunity to share their experiences and skills with students. In some courses it may even be appropriate to use whole communities as resources whom students can visit to gain practical experience or to gather data or information. If you use communities and their institutions in this way have you considered them as a resource which could be developed even further? Involving resource people in the planning of fieldwork and its supervision, consulting community leaders about needs which might be serviced by students, and seeking feedback on the performance of the students in the field, are all methods which can be used to involve people as valuable learning resources. If they are made to feel an important part of the educational program then they are more likely to be an effective and reuseable resource.

FACILITIES

Activity:
Think of the facilities that are available in your school which might be helpful in your teaching. It may be worthwhile making a list. Try to think a little further afield than the usual laboratories, classrooms and clinics. Are there other facilities that you have not used, or perhaps are not aware of? Investigate a little, ask your colleagues and students.

Feedback:
An important part of the teacher's job is to investigate and become familiar with the facilities that are available. Many facilities are underused because teachers are not aware of their existence, or are not familiar with their use. On the other hand, many facilities lie idle because 'they seemed a good idea at the time' and were purchased or built without adequate consultation with teaching staff to determine their real usefulness. Inadequate provision for equipment maintenance is another mistake which frequently limits the potential of many facilities. If the overhead projector always blows a globe when teachers want to use it they soon learn to do without.
    Even if you are aware of all of the facilities available to you are you sure you are using them to their best advantage? It is possible, for example, that some classrooms do not have fixed seating and that seats could be rearranged so that you could plan a group discussion instead of a lecture on suitable topics. Are you allowing students

sufficient free time to make good use of the library as a self-directed learning tool or do you just prescribe readings from a few tried and true textbooks? Chakrabarty (1983) has provided guidelines for the use of libraries as information resources for nurse education. Imaginative use of existing facilities may be the solution to many of your teaching problems.

LEARNING MATERIALS

The bulk of this chapter is devoted to learning materials, not because they are more important than people or other facilities, but because they are not specifically limited by your situation and so some general principles can be discussed which apply to most teaching and learning contexts.

Activity:
What learning materials do you currently use? Are there any others that you would like to try but have not yet used? If so, why haven't you used them?

Feedback:
The variety of learning materials you can use is limited only by your imagination and the facilities you have available. The biggest problem in using learning resources is learning how to choose the most appropriate ones from the vast range of options that are available. The larger your budget the bigger the problem of choosing. Basically, the two options are to buy or to make your own. Only you can make the decision but bear in mind that the most important consideration is whether the materials which are purchased commercially turn out to be inappropriate because of differences in terminology or common practice or because they are pitched at the wrong level for the learners. A good rule to follow is **never buy before you try.** Catalogue entries may be very misleading. You should be able to obtain catalogues of available nursing materials from your local professional association or from the librarian of

your school library.

Making your own materials

Teachers often find it is more suitable to make their own materials because in that way they can be sure that the materials provide exactly the information which is appropriate to their particular classes. Most teachers who have decided to make their own, either with or without the assistance of a technical production unit, have found the task to be very time consuming. However, it is time well spent for a number of reasons. Firstly, what you produce will be used by many students, perhaps over many years so that the efficiency and cost benefit is high. Secondly, in the process of clarifying what you want to include in the learning materials you might find that you gain a better insight into the topic and are able to better plan other aspects of your teaching. Thirdly, if the materials successfully replace some repetitive aspects of teaching then you are free to give more individual attention to students, or to engage the class in higher level activities such as problem solving and discussion.

If you have decided to make your own materials the rest of this chapter provides some basic guidance. There are many books (for example Brown, Lewis & Harcleroad, 1973 and Tindall, Collins & Reid, 1973) which can provide more detailed advice if you require it and do not have technical production personnel to help you.

Activity:
The following is a list of the types of materials or media most commonly used in nursing education:

Handouts, printed notes and texts
Drawings, graphs and diagrams
Photographs, 35mm slides
Films
Videotapes
Models of real objects or simulations
Real objects, people or events.

The materials or media are listed in that particular order for a specific reason. Can you explain why they have been placed in that order?

Feedback:
   They are in that order because those media at
the top of the list are furthest away from reality
while those at the bottom of the list represent
reality itself or a close approximation. Perhaps we
should clear up a small problem of definition.
Medium is used in this context to mean the methods
used for transmission of a message, for example
television is a medium, tape slide programs are
media. Materials are the programs, photographs,
diagrams etc. which make up the messages which are
transmitted via the various media.
   If you are intending to produce your own
materials your first decision will be which medium
to employ. To a certain extent your decision will
be influenced by what you have available but beyond
that your decision should be based on the learning
objectives, in other words on the nature of the
learning that you intend the materials to help the
students achieve. As a rule of thumb:

**If the learning involves understanding or
comprehension of knowledge or relationships between
parts of systems or objects then simple resources
such as diagrams with class notes or handouts will
be most useful.**

**If the learning involves recognition of real
objects or events then real objects or events must
be used and practice in discrimination provided.**

**Reality or media closely resembling reality may
present information which is initially too complex
for effective learning.**

**For some skills and knowledge learning it may be
most effective to use a series of media which
progressively increase the level of realism once
students have learned to cope with the basic
understanding, recognition and discrimination which
will allow them to perform appropriately.**

   For example, if students are learning to
manage venous stasis ulcers then they will be
required to understand the basic structure of the
lesion to recognise a stasis ulcer and perhaps
discriminate it from a squamous cell carcinoma, and
to be able to effectively carry out wound toilet

and dressings. The most appropriate medium for teaching the basic structure of the ulcer may be a simple chalkboard diagram of a cross-section of the ulcer demonstrating its shape and the layers of the skin which are ulcerated. Helping students to discriminate amongst different types of ulcers may be achieved by showing numerous examples of ulcers and discussing their similarities and differences, however, this is likely to be difficult to do in the clinic or ward and so a more effective learning experience might consist of a classroom session in which students are shown 35mm slides and given practice in discriminating with ample opportunity for discussion and feedback. Learning to keep the ulcer clean and properly dressed can only be achieved in the real situation where students observe the procedure and are able to carry it out under supervision, however certain aspects of the skill can be practised in simulated conditions, for example using the sterile pack, applying dressings and bandages, and advising the patient on the proper after care and follow-up.

One more word of advice before we proceed – always choose the simplest and least expensive medium that will do the job to ensure that both you and the students enjoy maximum access to and benefit from the materials you have worked so hard to produce.

Activity:
At this point you will probably find it useful to pause and give some thought to the type of learning resources you would like to produce. A good starting point is to identify an area of your teaching which has been problematic for some reason. Analyse the problem, would it be helped by better use of learning resources? What is the nature of the learning and learning objectives for the problem area? What type of medium would be an effective resource and why?

Feedback:
Keep this activity in mind as you work through the rest of this chapter. Some of the examples given, and the media and materials described might

be relevant to your specific problem or at least might provide you with leads to follow up in other areas.

Handouts and course notes

Handouts or course notes are particularly useful for topics for which there are no suitable textbooks available. Handouts are sometimes given to students, and sometimes sold to cover the costs of printing; whichever method your school uses the costs of printing or duplication are sufficiently high that it is worth making sure that the notes you provide are valuable. A good summary of points to consider in the design of instructional text has been provided by Hartley (1978).

Teachers often ask when handouts should be given to students. There is no simple answer to this question because, as with many of the questions addressed in this book, it all depends on the purpose of the handouts and their role in helping the students to learn. The first important thing to mention is that there are many different types of handout with many different purposes, for example handouts may be any one or a combination of the following:

full transcripts of lectures
summaries or lists of important aspects of the lecture
copies of graphs or diagrams used in the class
key points of the lesson phrased as headings or questions with space left for students to fill in their own notes
lists of objectives for the course or lesson
information or details relating to logistics of courses.

Full transcripts of lectures or complete printed notes may be useful if students have no access to a library or textbooks but they are also costly to produce and research has indicated that students learn better from notes they have written themselves than from complete notes provided by the teacher. (Hartley & Davies, 1978).

In general the most educationally useful type of handouts are the ones which provide the structure or outline of the lesson and some stimulus such as questions to help the students organise their thinking and notetaking during the class (Brown & Tomlinson, 1980). Diagrams and important sketches can also be provided to ensure that students have an accurate record of the information but do not have to waste valuable class time copying it down. Diagrams can be incomplete so that students are required to make some notes in relation to them, perhaps labelling anatomical structures or making interpretations of graphs. A framework handout of this type which invites student participation to complete it ensures that students remain attentive throughout the class and are aware of where the class is taking them (see Figure 6.1).

Figure 6.1: EXAMPLE OF A FRAMEWORK HANDOUT

Course: Maternal and Child Health
Topic: Normal Milestones

At the end of this class you should be able to identify the normal milestones in the development of an infant.

What are the parameters by which milestones are measured?

How are normal criteria for those milestones developed?

What are the normal values of the parameters employed at specified ages?

What are the main causes of failure to thrive in this society?

How would you interpret this graph of weight for age for an infant? (Insert graph here)

Activity: Design a handout for a class that you teach. Make sure that it:
  a) provides students with the objectives and structure of the class
  b) encourages student involvement with the material presented both in the class and in the handout

c) includes any information such as dosages, technical terms, graphs or complex diagrams which students must know but which they might copy incorrectly into their notes if pressed for time.

Feedback:
    The best feedback on your handout will come from your students. Try using it next time you teach that topic and ask the students for their opinions and suggestions.

Photographs

    The types of photographs most commonly used in teaching are 35mm slides. Printing of good quality black and white photographs in booklets is relatively simple but of limited value in clinical conditions where colour is an important part of the information. Coloured slides can provide excellent resolution of detail and realistic colour to make identification of clinical or histological detail relatively simple. Most teachers will have access to a medical illustration unit in a hospital or an audio-visual production unit in their school so it is not the purpose here to go into production detail which is readily available elsewhere. For the interested teacher a good general introduction to photography can be found in 'The Joy of Photography' by the editors of the Eastman Kodak Company (1980). The Eastman Kodak Company has also produced a series of technical pamphlets dealing with scientific photography and the educational use of 35mm slides. Your local Kodak representative should be able to provide details. (For more specifically clinical educational applications see Garrick, 1978; Ewan, 1981).

Activity:
Do you use photographs in your teaching? What is the main purpose for which you use them? Have you considered using them for other purposes?

Feedback:

Most teachers use slides in lectures at one time or another to illustrate some conditions or procedure which cannot be brought into the classroom. Some teachers use slides as reminders of what they wanted to say in the lecture or as alternatives to writing or drawing on the blackboard. All of these are reasonable uses if the slides are properly designed and presented, although lists, diagrams and graphs are probably more effectively and cheaply presented using the overhead projector. In brief, the most appropriate reasons for using slides in a lecture or class are:

1. To present the real appearance of a person, a clinical condition or an object when it is not possible to bring the real person, condition or object into the classroom.
2. Photographs are always available to fit in with your timetable, suitable patients to illustrate your topic may not be.
3. Many patients have atypical or incomplete manifestations of clinical features and therefore may be a source of confusion to students in the initial phase of learning about the topic. Your photographs have been chosen by you because they show exactly what you want them to show and they eliminate confusing extra information.
4. Photographs can be used to enhance the important aspects of which you want to make students aware. For example you can use close-ups of particular conditions or pieces of equipment.
5. Features demonstrated in photographs are more freely able to be discussed and used for repetitive practice in recognition than they would be if the same features were being demonstrated in a clinic or ward situation.

So far we have talked about using slides in lectures or classes but slides have an additional context in which they have proven very useful and that is in self-instruction. Self-instructional programs have been widely used in health professions education over the past fifteen years (Ewan 1982). The most valuable contribution of such self-instructional programs is their ability to allow students to proceed at their own pace through material which has visual as well as verbal knowledge components. Such programs can be used as remedial materials for students who have fallen behind in specific aspects of class work, or as enrichment materials for students who are making better than average progress or as mastery based learning materials for all students who proceed systematically through a planned series of learning units, moving to each new unit following mastery of the material in the preceding units. The theoretical basis of mastery learning has been discussed in Chapter 3.

The basic steps in producing a self-instructional program will be dealt with later in this chapter.

A variant of 35mm slides which has also become popular is the microfiche card similar to those used for library catalogues. The advantage of microfiche reproduction of slides is that once the master microfiche card has been produced multiple copies containing between 49 and 60 colour photographs can be produced very cheaply. It is possible, using microfiche systems and portable microfiche viewers, to provide every student with copies of cards and accompanying notes for home study. A good discussion of the use of microfiche in teaching neuroanatomy is given by Watson (1982), and in biomedical education in general by Garfield (1980).

Remember that a photograph is only as good as the teacher who uses it.

- Plan your photographs to make sure that they contain relevant and important information.
- Ensure that slides are clearly visible from the back row of the classroom (for details see Kodak S-22 and S-24). If you can read a slide without a magnifier, people in the back row will probably be able to read it on the screen.
  Never photograph tables or graphs out of books, the printing is invariably too crowded, small and indistinct for legibility when projected. If necessary use a printed graph but cut the labelling from the axes and redo it in larger letters. Be sure to check your copyright laws first!
- Framing is important. Avoid unnecessary background detail by placing the object to be photographed in front of a plain screen. Make

sure that the information you want to show in your photograph does not have competition from equally interesting but irrelevant information in other parts of the photograph. How often have you been subjected to a presentation where the speaker projects a complex table or diagram and says 'now I want you just to pay attention to this part here in the corner'?

- When using close-up (for example of a skin lesion) remember that there are few clues in the photograph to orient the viewer. How big is it? Where on the body is it situated? This problem can be solved by using a context shot before, and possibly after the close up.
- Another aspect of this problem of context is scale. How big is the object in the photograph? The viewer has no way of knowing unless there is something of known size in the photograph to compare it with.
- Labelling of photographs used for slides can be helpful especially if the slides are to be used as part of self-instructional packages, but keep labelling to a minimum. Too many labels can divert attention from the important content of the photograph. When you are using the slide in a lecture presentation labels in the photograph are more distracting and you would do better to avoid their use and use a pointer instead to indicate specific aspects of the photograph.
- Last but certainly not least remember that you are part of the audio-visual display. Never try to compete with your own slides. Vision is a more powerful sense than hearing. If there is a conflict between the messages presented to the students' eyes and the messages presented to their ears they are more likely to attend to what they see than what they hear. In practical terms when you have finished describing or discussing a particular slide and wish to move on to talk about something else switch off the projector until you are ready to talk about the next slide.

The overhead projector

In the past twenty years overhead projectors have gained a place in every classroom. Some teachers use them merely as a substitute for the chalkboard but their potential is much greater than this.

Activity:
List the special advantages of the overhead projector that make it particularly helpful in your teaching. How do you use it?

Feedback:
One of the biggest advantages of the overhead projector is that it does not need to be used in a darkened room so that students are able to take notes without difficulty. A second significant advantage is that the teacher is able to face the class while writing on transparencies, rather than having to turn his or her back as is the case when writing on the chalkboard. A third major advantage is that transparencies can be prepared beforehand and used as a planning device for the class or lecture. Several transparencies can be built up in sequence one on top of the other to show progressive amounts of detail. This is a particularly useful facility in Anatomy for example, where the teacher can use a drawing of the bony skeleton of the limb and then an overlay which puts the muscles into position on that skeleton and then overlays of the vascular and nerve supply to the limb. Overlays can be used for progressive build up of any complex diagram so that students are helped to understand pieces of the whole and their relationship to one another with your guidance rather than being presented with a complete diagram and having to find their way around it. A related strategy for effective use of the overhead projector is called progressive disclosure. Progressive disclosure is most useful when you have a list of items to discuss. If you project the whole list students will copy it down immediately and miss what you are saying in relation to the first one or two items. If you attach the transparency to a cardboard frame, flaps of paper or cardboard can be attached to the frame and as each item is discussed, its corresponding flaps can be turned back to reveal that item.
Student participation in class can be enhanced by the overhead projector. Since transparencies are

easy to produce, groups of students can be given problems to solve or issues to discuss and asked to return to the class with a summary of their work on an overhead transparency for sharing with the rest of the class. Overhead projectors can also be used to project the shapes of solid objects such as surgical instruments and they are effective for showing gross details of radiographs or even computerized axial tomography scans. At a pinch the overhead projector can be used to project images on microfilm or microfiche cards. There are many ways to use the overhead projector to great effect in education; it is worth experimenting a little in your subject to make sure that you are using it to its full potential.

A word about producing transparencies. Your local distributor of projectors and projector products can probably provide you with a great deal of information about various approaches to producing overhead projection transparencies. The cheapest approach is to use a continuous roll of acetate film which can be attached to the projector and rolled across the screen as you write. Transparencies can be prepared beforehand on the continuous roll however most teachers find this very inconvenient and prefer to use single sheet transparencies. Single sheet transparencies are of two basic types, 'write-on' and heat sensitive.

Heat sensitive transparencies are available in a variety of formats which make possible various special colour effects, for example red image on a black background or blue image on a clear background. These transparencies tend to be more expensive and apart from their dramatic effect have little educational advantage. Black image on a clear or faint blue background gives the most legible effect and is most commonly used. A master is prepared by typewriter (only very large typefaces are legible) or by hand (using a pencil) and is passed through a thermal copier with the heat sensitive film. The carbon image absorbs heat and causes an image to appear on the film. Printed diagrams, graphs, carbon image photocopies of monochrome photographs and print can all be transferred to overhead transparency using this process. Remember that the original must be made using a substance such as carbon which can absorb heat, ordinary ball point pen will not produce an

173

image. Plain paper copier manufacturers also market overhead transparencies which can be used in their machines making it possible to produce transparency copies as easily as paper copies.

'Write on' transparencies are simply acetate sheets which can be written on using a special overhead projection pen, although beware, some acetate sheets have a right and wrong side. If you are having trouble writing on the sheet try the other side.

The basic rules of legibility apply to overhead transparencies as they do to 35mm slides. Normal typewriter print or print from books is too small, even the IBM Orator 'golfball' type is too small to be seen clearly in the average lecture room. Neat handprinting is preferable if you do not have access to a lettering machine or one of the special typewriters that produce large print. A good rule of thumb is that the transparency will be legible when projected if it can be read with the naked eye at a distance of two metres. Once again do not be tempted to copy graphs or tables from books, the students will not be able to read the print. Photocopy the graph, cut off the labelling and printing and use just the graph to make a new original, relabelling by hand or with a lettering machine, and then make your transparency. Most tables taken from books contain more information than you probably need in the class so it is worth the effort to summarise the information, including only the important aspects on a transparency that can be easily seen from the back of the class.

Television

We have chosen to deal here with television rather than film because most teachers in modern schools have greater access to video-production facilities than to film production facilities. The ease of inhouse production and the immediacy of videotape playback has elevated television to the pre-eminent position among educational media which can demonstrate motion. Commercially produced educational films are still available and have their place if the desire is to demonstrate high resolution motion photography in a topic which is sufficiently important to justify the expense of high quality film production. For most educational purposes however, videotape (actually cassette these days and videodisc more recently) is quite sufficient and cheaper to produce or purchase.

Activity:
In the topics that you teach what are the main potential uses for videotape?
Is there any particular approach that you would like to try? What facilities do you have for making your own videotape productions?

Feedback:
The features of video which set it apart from other colour motion media are the ability to obtain immediate replay with no need for development of the film, the reusability of tape or cassette which makes it economical for classroom use, and the ease of inhouse production due to high resolution portable equipment which has few special needs for lighting or sound reproduction. Acceptable videotapes can be made in normal classroom or clinic conditions. The packaging of the tape in videocassette format and the simplicity of use of the playback equipment means that videocassette is a convenient library resource which can be easily used by students as a self-instructional medium. Large screen television monitors also make it possible to use videocassette or tape in lecture or classroom situations.

The potential for television in biomedical and nursing education is vast. On the one hand it has great value in demonstrating clinical conditions and procedures which have a strong visual element and which cannot always be conveniently observed in real situations and on the other hand it represents the perfect tool for providing feedback to students on their skill development both in manual and interpersonal areas. Used for this latter purpose it enables students to view their own performance and in discussion with peers or teachers to systematically analyse the process and identify areas for improvement. For examples of television used in this way see Kagan (1980), Ryan-Merritt (1982). For general information on the use of instructional television see Schramm (1972) and for its use in biomedical education see Guest-Lee (1979) and Durbridge & Gale (1980).

175

Some teachers have the time and facilities to produce their own videotapes, some have access to good quality relevant programs which have been bought or borrowed from elsewhere. A reminder of what was said earlier in this chapter about using programs produced elsewhere: **it is important to view the programs before you use them with your class to ensure that the content and approach is appropriate for your students.** Cultural, language or technical differences in both films and videotapes may even interfere with student learning rather than assist it. Remember that if you are using the program in class you have control over it. If one segment is of particular value then show only that segment. If some parts require additional comment or explanation stop the tape and discuss the point with the class, replay selected segments to reinforce the message or to ensure that students have understood. Students gain more from a program when the teacher views it with them and interacts with the medium as part of the lesson rather than an extra activity. Similarly video or other programs used as self-instructional materials are more effective and more popular with students if teachers make it clear where the programs belong in the overall context of the teaching and learning. Media and materials should be integral parts of teaching and learning not optional or entertaining extras.

The following section describes a method for producing videotapes as self-instructional materials. The principles, however, also apply to the design of any program used for educational purposes and the same sequence of steps could be followed in the production of film, tape-slide programs, tape-booklets or even instructional booklets which incorporate illustrations.

Designing self-instructional materials

The flow chart in Figure 6.2 provides an outline of the steps through which you can proceed to produce an instructional television program. You can also modify that flow chart and apply it to the production of an instructional program using any other medium. To enlarge a little on each step begin by asking yourself the following:

1.   Who will view the program?

2. <u>What do you want the program to do?</u>
    Is it to provide information which is
    otherwise not available to students?
    Is it to demonstrate a skill that students
    must learn?
    Is it to act as a trigger to stimulate
    discussion or attitude change?

3. <u>Based on your answers to these questions write
    an outline</u> of what you want to cover in the
    program. A few hints based on the conditions
    for learning discussed in Chapter 3:
    Providing information
    -   design 'advance organisers'
    -   identify the key concepts to be
        learned and map their relationship to
        each other
    -   sequence the concepts
    -   design case studies and problems to
        present the concepts
    -   provide ample opportunities for
        practice, self-testing and student
        involvement with the material.

    Demonstrating skills
    -   analyse the skill into components
    -   demonstrate total skill, then compo-
        nent skills, then total skill again
    -   allow for practice
    -   choose a camera angle which will
        place the viewer in the position of
        the person performing the skill.

    Triggering discussion or attitude change
    -   create scenarios with which the
        viewer can identify and about which
        he or she may have some attitude
        already
    -   introduce elements which challenge
        likely existing attitudes and promote
        some cognitive or emotional conflict
        in the viewer
    -   keep it short and provocative
    -   make it relevant to the topic under
        discussion
    -   end with a question - stated or
        implied
    -   allow opportunities for resolution by
        providing ample time for discussion.

177

4. <u>Plan the program</u>. Arrange the content outline in a sequence which is suitable for helping your students to understand the message. This step is made easier by the 'storyboard' approach in which cards are sketched and scripted for each new idea to be introduced, and are arranged in sequence to form the program. Use the storyboard to plan the 'shots' that you will need and specify the technical details for the production crew, for example close-ups and camera angles.

5. <u>Write the script</u> - keep sentences brief and to the point, keep language simple and avoid repeating yourself. Check the storyboard to make sure that components of the script are linked to the relevant visuals. Insert problems or questions for students to answer.

6. <u>Produce visual materials</u> such as graphs or charts, and organize any other resources such as patients that you will need.

7. <u>Liaise with others involved in the production</u> - 'talent', technical crew and design staff and rehearse if necessary.

8. <u>Make the videorecording</u> (or in the case of other media, arrange for appropriate photography, studio-recording, printing etc.)

9. <u>Pilot test the finished product</u> by showing it to your colleagues and a sample of the students for whom it was designed and asking for specific feedback on aspects which could be improved. You might also wish to consult colleagues and students at an earlier stage in production such as the storyboard or script.

The following are some specific points to attend to in television production:

Action - Television is a motion medium so you should try to get some action. Have your 'talent' (students, teachers, patients) doing things - demonstrating a technique or talking to each other. When there is nothing for them to do switch to a shot of something that they

are talking about. Avoid the 'talking head' -
lengthy shots of someone talking to the
camera.

Technical Crew - The technical crew (if you are
lucky enough to have one) needs to be briefed
completely about what you are trying to
achieve with your program. They can advise
about the best shots to get your message
across. If you have a producer work closely
with him or her to plan special effects,
camera work, editing, inclusion of graphics,
close ups.

Design staff - Do not underestimate the planning
and time necessary for the preparation of
graphics such as title cards, graphs, tables,
illustrations and demonstration specimens.
Good communication between the teacher and the
designer, photographer or artist is essential.

If you are fortunate enough to have such
facilities make sure you use them to their best
potential by putting sufficient time into the
design of educationally sound programs. If yours is
a one-man or one-woman show you can still produce
very acceptable programs if you are prepared to run
through them a few times and learn from your
mistakes.

FIGURE 6.2: FLOW CHART FOR DESIGNING
SELF-INSTRUCTIONAL MATERIALS.

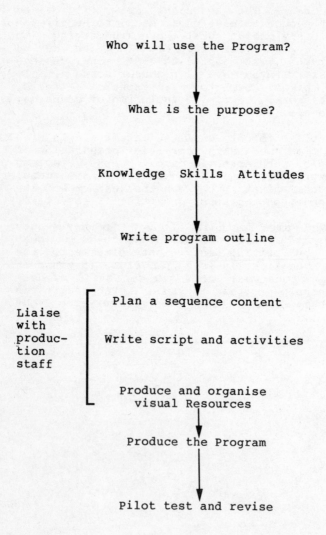

Who will use the Program?

What is the purpose?

Knowledge Skills Attitudes

Write program outline

Liaise
with
produc-
tion
staff

Plan a sequence content

Write script and activities

Produce and organise
visual Resources

Produce the Program

Pilot test and revise

Figure 6.3: APPRAISAL FORM

		Satis- factory	Unsatis- factory
A.	**TECHNICAL QUALITY**		
	1. Sound-track (if applicable)	....	....
	2. Quality of narrator's voice	....	....
	3. Appropriateness of illustrations	....	....
B.	**CONTENT QUALITY**		
	1. Accuracy	....	....
	2. Appropriateness to level of students	....	....
	3. Relevance to local conditions	....	....
	4. Appropriate organization of content	....	....
C.	**EDUCATIONAL QUALITY**		
	1. Aims of the material stated	....	....
	2. Content communicated efficiently	....	....
	3. Sequence logical	....	....
	4. Presentation to maintain interest	....	....
	5. Appropriate pacing	....	....
	6. Visuals and commentary complement each other	....	....
	7. Review of major points	....	....
	8. Duration of program	....	....

Activity:
Refer to the activity on page 165 where you decided what types of materials you want to produce. Follow the steps in Figure 6.2 and produce a draft of the program. Ask your students and colleagues for feedback. The appraisal form in Figure 6.3 is typical of the types of forms used to appraise materials for their educational usefulness. You could use it or a variation as a tool for obtaining useful feedback on your instructional program.

Simulations

The variety of available models and simulations is very broad, ranging from three-dimensional synthetic models of objects or parts of the body through computerised problem solving exercises or educational games.

The purpose behind all models and simulations is the same. They are intended to provide a means for students to learn new skills without risk to themselves or others and with the maximum opportunity for guided practice and feedback in a situation which closely resembles reality. Role play, a very useful simulation method in nursing education has already been discussed in Chapter 4. The use of educational games in nursing has been well described by Hope (1983) and general developments in the area have been summarised by Megarry (1979).

Two common physical simulations seen in nursing education are pelvic models for demonstration of the birth canal and cardio-pulmonary resuscitation models. Generally speaking those models which most closely resemble reality are also the most expensive. It is important when you are using such models in teaching to point out to students those ways in which they do differ from reality.

Other types of simulations help students to develop thinking skills rather than manual skills. Simulations which require students to analyse a clinical situation and solve a problem can be developed using either simple paper and pencil techniques or sophisticated computer programs. The methods you choose will depend on your resources, however once again the general principles can be applied across the range of simulations.

Barrows & Tamblyn (1980, p.164) have described the development of Portable Patient Problem Packs, variants on the same theme are Problem Boxes, or Patient Management Problems (Hunt, 1982). The formats differ mainly in the way information is presented to the student and the ways in which students respond to that information, making diagnostic and management choices. When students make correct choices they are allowed to move on through the programs, when they make incorrect choices they are given feedback and asked to choose other options. The least sophisticated forms employ limited options which are chosen by students in response to questions, and feedback which is revealed by various types of chemical print development. The most sophisticated forms consist of branching computer programs which can simulate real time patient encounters, allow considerable latitude for student responses and provide detailed feedback to students on their progress (Kirchoff & Holzemer, 1979). Simulations of this type are used not only for teaching purposes but also as assessment tools. Sweeney, O'Malley & Freeman (1982) have described the development of a computer simulation to evaluate the clinical performance of nursing students in a paper which is instructive for teachers who are contemplating using microcomputers for either skill development or assessment.

For those of you who are not yet ready to take on computer simulations a feasible and effective alternative is the **Problem Box.** Depending upon the clinical problem you wish to simulate, the problem box could include:

1.   A card describing the clinical scenario and the patient involved.
2.   Samples of relevant clinical material for students to interpret, for example temperature and blood pressure charts, photographs of the patient's appearance, nursing notes from the previous shift.
3.   A series of actions that the nurse could take to analyse the nursing problems, each written on a separate card (feedback as to the appropriateness of each action should be

written on the back of the card).
4.   A further series of cards which could follow
     up details of each appropriate action and the
     results obtained.

For each step in the formation of a solution
to the problem the student must make a decision
about what information to seek, how to interpret
that information and what actions to take as a
result. Because the student must commit him or
herself to choosing cards from the available
options both the student and the teacher can see
whether the choice is relevant and therefore
whether the problem has been approached in an
effective and efficient manner. By assigning marks
to cards and adding or deducting for correct or
incorrect answers the problem box can even be used
as an assessment tool.

Activity:
Design a problem box or some other type of
simulation which you would use in your
teaching.

Feedback:
Check your simulation against the following
checklist:
1.   Have you defined exactly what the
     simulation will help students to be able
     to do?
2.   Does the simulation provide a realistic
     problem or context which closely resembles
     one in which your students will have to
     work?
3.   Does the simulation provide enough
     practice in making decisions and
     interpreting information?
4.   Does the simulation make the student
     responsible for the outcomes - is it clear
     that the outcomes are a result of the
     actions and judgements of the student?
5.   Does the simulation provide feedback to
     the student on how well the task is being
     performed in relation to standard
     criteria?
6.   Is the simulation non-threatening so that

the student is free to learn without fear of ridicule or harsh criticism?
7. Is the simulation easy to manage and economical to produce?

While this checklist will provide you with some guidance as to the likely effectiveness of your simulation it is absolutely necessary that you test your prototype simulation with a group of students before producing it in quantity. A bad simulation runs considerable risk of confusing students and producing the opposite educational effect to the one that you intended.

SUMMARY

The best resources are those which you have chosen because they can help your students to learn what they must know. You should therefore, choose resources which
- are appropriate for the level of students and the type of learning they must achieve,
- present the main message clearly, and are free from distraction by irrelevant details,
- encourage the students to be actively involved with the material rather than merely passive receivers of information,
- are technically well produced, accurate and educationally sound,
- are able to be easily and confidently used by you and your students.

Chapter 7

ASSESSING LEARNING

Developments and trends in nursing education discussed elsewhere in this book have been accompanied by a critical examination of assessment of student learning. Traditional assumptions have been questioned and innovative approaches to assessing many aspects of performance have been, and continue to be, developed. Assessment is no longer viewed as an unidimensional test of student ability but rather as a multidimensional part of the learning process. Devising methods for assessment which contribute to the students' learning has become a major component of the teacher's job.

When you have completed this chapter you should be able to identify the purposes of student assessment, to choose assessment strategies appropriate to those purposes and to plan and implement effective assessment procedures.

It will be useful to begin by clarifying three terms which are often used interchangeably - assessment, evaluation and examination. For the purposes of this chapter 'assessment' is taken to mean the processes by which teachers attempt to gauge students' progress and learning; assessment may or may not involve quantifying that progress in terms of marks or grades. 'Evaluation' is reserved for the broader process of determining the effectiveness of the education students are receiving; assessment will contribute to evaluation but so may other processes such as observations of teaching, interviews, and opinion surveys. 'Examination' refers to the formal mechanisms by which assessment is sometimes accomplished.

PURPOSES OF ASSESSMENT

As with most educational planning, the
planning of assessment requires that you decide
what you are trying to achieve before you embark on
your planning exercise. Too often assessments are
planned from the other direction - teachers start
from the point of planning assessments to fit with
the traditional pattern of their school, for
example end of term examinations or final
examinations. A more rational starting point is
from the consideration of the purposes of the
assessment.

Activity:
Think of the assessments which your students
undertake. Make a list of the assessments, the
times at which they are carried out and the
main purposes for which they are intended.

Feedback:
As a minimum you have probably listed term
tests whose marks contribute towards final grades
given the student, and end of year or final
examinations whose marks determine whether students
will be permitted to progress to the next stage of
the course or to graduate or be registered to
practise.

Until a few years ago this would have been an
average schedule of assessments in many nursing
schools. It fulfils the first main purpose of
assessment : to allow you to certify students as
competent (in theory at least, but more about that
later). These assessments have been called
**'summative' because they represent the aggregate or
final result of student learning.** Such a limited
schedule however, neglects the other important
purpose of assessment which is to help students to
learn. Of course it may motivate students to learn,
but that is not the same as ensuring that their
learning is useable, and lasting (see Chapter 3).
Assessments used as a method to guide learning in

progress have been called **'formative' because, by providing feedback on performance they help the students to form or shape their learning in desired directions.**

Assessments, used as contributors to learning can achieve the following purposes:

1. They can be more reliable in certifying competence if they are employed over a wide range of time and experience throughout the students' learning career to ensure that students are mastering the learning objectives as they proceed.

2. They can help students to determine how well they are progressing and to estimate how much more work and in which areas they should concentrate to reach an acceptable criterion.

3. They can help the teacher to identify individual learning needs and to suggest remedial action.

4. They can provide practice for students in self- and peer assessment, skills they will need when they are practising professional nurses.

5. They can encourage students to keep up to date with class work, rather than adopting the very ineffective strategy of 'cramming' at the last minute.

6. They can help the teacher to determine how effective the course is.

The main thrust behind all of these purposes is that assessment can be used throughout the learning as a diagnostic aid and a source of feedback to both teacher and student. Contrast this with the more traditional approach where assessment took place at the end of the course or unit of learning, where feedback was given to the student in the form of grades or marks and where the student had no opportunity or even specific information to enable her to make good the deficits in learning. In view of the fact that pass marks for such examinations were invariably considerably less than 100% we can assume that significant numbers of nurses were able to graduate with significant gaps in their knowledge and skills, and worse still, no information about what those gaps were.

In response to this realisation, the most significant recent shift in philosophy of assessment in the health professions has been the shift away from norm-referenced assessment towards criterion-referenced assessment.

Activity:
If you are familiar with the terms norm-reference and criterion-referenced, take a few minutes to draw up a table which contrasts their main features. If you are not familiar with those terms proceed straight to the feedback for this activity.

Feedback:
Norm-referenced assessment is the familiar process by which students are given marks and then graded according to their performance in comparison with other students in the class. Often, fairly arbitrary cut-off points are adopted for pass/fail or the award of honours. For example an A grade might represent marks between 85% and 100%, a B grade might represent 70% to 84%, a C grade 55% to 69% and a fail might be less than 55%. Problems arise in this system from time to time when, for example, a whole class performs less well than expected, perhaps due to the characteristics of the examination, or the teaching, or the students. In any case faculty are faced with the decision to either fail a high number of students and award less A grades or to shift the pass mark downwards. The latter is a regrettable choice in the health professions where schools are accountable for the safety of patients served by their graduates, however it has been known to happen. The term 'norm-referenced' is derived from the fact that a graph of the distribution of student marks in examinations is usually normally distributed with the bulk of students achieving in the middle range and smaller numbers tailing off at each end of the curve as failures or distinctions.

189

Plainly translated, norm-referenced certifying examinations tell us that the faculty are satisfied to produce a small percentage of excellent students, a small percentage of failures and a majority of mediocre or barely competent students. After all how certain can we be that the student who scores 56% and passes is more competent than the student who scores 54% and fails? The main justification for accepting this state of affairs has been that student ability is normally distributed and that examination performance reflects that innate ability and is therefore not amenable to teaching intervention.

Criterion-referenced assessment, in contrast, draws on the philosophy of mastery learning discussed in Chapter 3, in which it is suggested that, given appropriate teaching intervention, almost all students can achieve a high level of mastery - certainly in a tertiary level course in which students have been selected on the basis of their ability to begin with. Criterion-referenced assessment does not depend on comparisons among students, but on the extent to which each individual student is able to achieve the criterion set. Under ideal conditions the implication is that no students will fail and that all students will achieve 100% or very close to it. The normal curve no longer applies, and faculty who embark on this approach may find difficulty with their colleagues who equate high pass rates with 'too easy exams' or 'soft options' and who may demand that students be graded for administrative purposes. Krumme (1975) has provided a good summary of the case for criterion-referenced measurement in nursing.

A summary comparison table of the two forms of assessment should include the following elements:

TABLE 7.1 :   COMPARISON OF NORM & CRITERION-
REFERENCED ASSESSMENT

Non-referenced assessment	Criterion-referenced assessment
Compares students with each other	Compares students with criterion
Easy to grade students	Difficult to grade students
Must provide uniform conditions of time, place & items	Uniformity not necessary - may be tested at any time
Assumes learning rates are equal	Allows for individual differences in rates of learning
Does not require definition of objectives & performance criteria	Specific learning objectives and performance criteria essential
Students unsure of what to learn	Students know exactly what is expected of them
Maintains dependence on teacher as arbiter of success	Develops self-direction and skills in self-assessment
Might not ensure competence in essential areas	Ensures competence in essential areas
Does not provide specific feedback on mastery	Provides specific feedback on mastery of essential areas
Encourages competition between students	Encourages cooperation between students

You may now be convinced (if you weren't to begin with) that criterion-referenced assessment is a desirable goal for teachers in nursing to work towards. You might not be able to change all your assessment procedures overnight so you should concentrate on identifying those areas of your subject which will most benefit from adoption of criterion-referenced and mastery-based learning experiences. Remember that, since students are not going to be graded on their performance in comparison with each other, you do not have to be concerned over secrecy of test items or providing uniform conditions to ensure fairness to every student. Each student is to be assessed individually on his or her merits and the conditions operating at the time of the assessment can be taken into account in deciding whether the student has achieved the criterion you would expect under those conditions. This means that criterion-referenced assessment can be an ongoing part of student learning wherever that occurs, and that feedback is available to the student as often as is necessary for the student to achieve the set criterion. Unfortunately, this very advantage also creates problems for the teacher and student if not handled correctly.

Activity:
What problems do you envisage or have you experienced in the implementation of criterion-referenced assessment incorporating mastery-based learning? What solutions could be applied to those problems?

Feedback:
Problems and solutions in criterion-referenced assessment
A frequent problem is that, since criterion-referenced assessment can occur throughout the term or throughout the year in the form of progressive or formative assessment to provide feedback on progress, students begin to feel overexamined and constantly under stess. This problem applies particularly if the progressive assessments contribute to overall grading or marks. The climate

which is essential for growth and skill development is lacking in situations where students fear revealing their uncertainties and deficiencies to their supervisors or tutors because they may be held against them in future assessments. Morgan, Luke and Herbert (1979) have pointed out that, especially in the clinical setting, students' achievement is too often evaluated while they are still learning. They advocate ensuring that teachers and students realise that there should be a time to learn and make mistakes which is distinct from the time to be evaluated. Simulations can be employed to ensure that the learning period of assessment is risk-free. Only when students have reached a satisfactory predetermined mastery criterion should they be assessed on their performance in the real situation and evaluated against the criteria for professional performance. Another variant of this solution is the establishment of a contract or understanding between students and supervisors which acknowledges the students' right to determine when assessment will take place. Students may be informally assessed by tutors or supervisors and provided with guidance and feedback on performance until the student, or the student and supervisor in conference, decide that the student is ready for formal assessment by another assessor. This strengthens the bond of trust and cooperation between student and supervisor and maximises the students' opportunities to achieve mastery.

Mastery learning and criterion-referenced assessment can be very time-consuming and administratively difficult, given the likelihood that there will be considerable variation in the time taken for some students to achieve the criterion level. Theoretically, students should have all the time and help that they need, however in the real world this is rarely possible and teachers usually have to make decisions, based on their experience, about the maximum amount of time that a student can be allowed to persevere. Students who are markedly out of step with their colleagues should probably be counselled about their level of motivation to become a nurse, or their personal problems which might be interfering with their learning efficiency. However, even within predetermined time limits, it is a challenging administrative exercise to ensure that all students are gainfully employed both before and after achieving mastery. Students who achieve mastery earlier can act as helpers to their colleagues, providing guidance and feedback and thus saving the teacher some time. This is usually a valuable experience for both students since they are developing skills in giving and receiving feedback from peers and the assistance given by one student to the other reinforces the 'teacher-student's' knowledge and skills. Alternatively, faster students can be advanced to the next criterion task or can be given extra activities or responsibilities to extend their mastery of the topic. This approach also provides one solution to the dilemma of grading - extra credits towards advanced grades can be earned by students who contract to undertake activities beyond the basic mastery level. An approach to contract grading in clinical evaluation has been described by Schoolcraft and Delaney (1982).

One of the biggest advantages of criterion-referenced assessment also proves to be one of the biggest problems for some teachers, and that is the necessity to develop clear objectives for learning upon which criteria can be based. This invariably presents a number of dilemmas. It is necessary to be fairly specific in defining such criteria otherwise they are useless - for example 'demonstrates appropriate nursing behaviour' is an example of a criterion performance which is open to a wide variety of interpretation and therefore unlikely to provide a reliable basis for assessment. A more specific behaviour might be 'demonstrates use of the nursing process in the approach to patient care'. A more specific criterion still would be 'demonstrates skills in assessing, planning, implementing and evaluating when offering nursing care to a hospitalised patient for whom she has been given responsibility'. Of course we can go further still and probably keep going for quite some time in spelling out specific criterion behaviours within each of those skill areas of assessing, planning, implementing and evaluating. The teacher's problem becomes one of knowing where to stop. One of the dangers of specifying criteria is that, as competences are broken down into more and more discrete subskills we tend to lose sight of the overall picture, so that we run the risk of assessing students on their ability to perform discrete observable skills rather than to deliver effective care to the whole patient. No one can give you the ideal answer to this dilemma of how specific to be in defining objectives and criteria because the need for specificity will clearly be greater in some circumstances than others. For example, junior nursing students will need more guidance about the component skills involved in phases of the nursing process, or in preparing a patient for surgery or in relating to bereaved relatives, however it can be assumed that senior students have mastered the basic skills and so assessment can be based on more holistic criteria such as the effective use of nursing process, the preparation, both physical and psychological, of patients for surgery and the empathic professional approach to bereaved relatives. At this level, according to Woolley (1977) 'Evaluation .... is making a subjective judgement about the meaningfulness of the whole, both from the parts that are measurable, and from those that must be assessed intuitively'. The point being that we must also assess those aspects of nursing care which are not so easily reduced to specific components of observable behaviour.

Chapter 2 has dealt, in some detail, with the process of defining learning objectives or outcomes. The remainder of this chapter will address the methods for translating those objectives into criteria for assessment.

METHODS OF ASSESSMENT

Planning the assessment program

Once you have decided whether you intend to use criterion-referenced or norm-referenced assessment and whether you intend to include formative as well as summative assessments in your program you must then begin to ask yourself exactly what you wish to assess and exactly what methods will best enable you to assess those learning outcomes.

Activity:
For the course that you teach how do you decide what to include in assessments? Include both formative and summative assessments in your considerations.

Feedback:
What to assess
It has been suggested that student learning can be divided into three categories (Abbatt, 1980):
1. MUST KNOW
2. SHOULD KNOW
3. NICE TO KNOW

Clearly, if you are interested in assessing student competence in essential criteria you will choose to assess the learning which is included in the 'must know' and also ideally, in the 'should know' categories. On the other hand, if your main purpose is to obtain a broad spread of marks which will allow you to grade and rank students you will probably want to include a number of items which assess 'nice to know' learning to sort out those students who have exceeded the basic requirements. There is nothing wrong with adopting this approach, ranking of students is often necessary in order to award prizes or make employment decisions; however 'nice to know' is no substitute for 'must know' and assessments in nursing should always ensure that essential performance criteria are assessed as an absolute minimum. Then if there is time, energy and reason enough, students can be given the opportunity to demonstrate how far beyond their basic mastery levels they have been able to progress. Unfortunately, some examiners still concentrate on asking obscure or 'nice to know' information at the expense of 'must know' in the interests of producing a 'good discriminating test' rather than a good measure of competence. To illustrate, in a norm-referenced test the most efficient item is one which only 50% of students answered correctly, this is the item on which the test score variance is largest. Small variance lowers estimates of item reliability and variability. On the other hand, in a criterion-referenced test the most efficient item is one which most students answered correctly (Kirby, 1977).

If your assessment is intended to test mastery of 'must know' objectives it naturally follows that students must know what those objectives are and therefore what they will be tested on. Some teachers object to this approach because they feel that students should not know what is going to be in the examination. Once again, this is an assumption which applies to norm-referenced assessments rather than criterion-referenced. If students are to be assessed on their mastery of set criteria there is no need for secrecy as there is if they are to be assessed for the purpose of ranking them against each other. Examinations are not supposed to trick or catch out the unprepared student, or to reward the student who is best able to 'psyche out' the hidden agenda of the teacher, but they are supposed to provide a fair assessment of how well the students have learned what they are supposed to have learned.

In summary then, if you are committed to the mastery philosophy your assessment will include at least all those knowledge, skills and attitudes which are considered to be essential learning for nursing competence. If you prefer to remain with norm-referenced assessment your assessment should provide a sample of the field of knowledge, both essential and non-essential, which will enable you to discriminate amongst students based on the broad spread of their marks.

Formative assessment has an important role in criterion-referenced assessment since it may be impossible to include all of the essential performances in a single examination or even series of examinations at the end of the term, or the year, or the course. Assessments of mastery can be offered at appropriate points throughout the learning period and can be recorded to contribute to the final certification of competence. For example, assessments at the completion of clinical attachment periods can be used in this way.

The following checklist will assist you in planning your assessment:

1. Select the 'must know' and 'should know'

objectives of your course.

2. Determine the knowledge, skills and attitudes components of those objectives.

3. Ensure that the level is appropriate - are you testing problem-solving or just recall of facts, are you testing skill components or holistic patient care?

4. Decide when would be the most appropriate time to assess each of these objectives. This will depend to a large extent on the structure of your course, but remember the importance of formative assessment and try to divide the course content into discrete units which can be conveniently followed by tests of mastery of the unit objectives.

5. Decide what type of assessment would be most appropriate for each objective, for example written tests can satisfactorily assess knowledge but procedural skills can only be effectively assessed in a clinical or simulated situation.

6. Within each type of assessment decide which format would best serve your purposes within your available resources, for example would your knowledge objectives be best assessed by multiple choice, essays, short answer questions or a combination of all?

7. Determine ways in which you will grade students if you require to do so. You could offer optional extra assessments or assignments, you could insert test items of greater difficulty, you could include some 'nice to know' objectives, you could determine weightings of marks on the basis of levels of objectives, or you could try offering students the opportunity to contract for higher grades.

8. Develop your assessment items or protocols and subject them to review by your colleagues. Do they meet the criteria for a good test - reliability, validity, feasibility? Will you need to train other assessors to ensure proper

application of the assessment?

9.   Check your final assessment program to ensure
     that all essential competences are represented
     and that you are assessing necessary higher
     order skills, attitudes and intellectual
     abilities rather than just knowledge.

**Remember that since all students aim to pass
examinations, assessments exert a powerful
influence on what students learn and the way they
learn. Make sure that your examination questions
are a good example of what you want the students to
learn. If you do not test for essential skills then
students are unlikely to bother to learn those
skills properly.**

Assessment Methods
     There is a large variety of assessment
methods, many of which you will be familiar with
and will have used on many occasions. Some newer
methods however, are worth a closer look and
perhaps some of the older methods you have been
using could be used more effectively. A number of
comprehensive books on assessment in general, and
assessment in the health professions and nursing
specifically are available (Adkins, 1974; Morgan &
Irby, 1978; Schneider, 1979; and Katz & Snow, 1980)
so it is intended in the following to provide an
overview of the major considerations in choosing
assessment methods with specific references for
more detailed aspects.

Activity:
The following are some of the 'must know'
objectives from your course. What method would
you use to assess performance in each area.

i)   Students must be able to recognise the
     clinical features of myocardial infarction.

ii) Students must be able to record an accurate
     history and assess the nursing care needs of a
     patient admitted to the coronary care unit.

iii) Students must be able to develop a nursing

199

plan for the care of a patient admitted to the coronary care unit.

iv)   Students must be able to correctly set up the cardiac arrest trolley.

v)   Students must be able to assist in the emergency management of a patient with cardiac arrest.

vi)   Students must demonstrate care and concern for the wellbeing of patients in their care and consideration for the needs of the relatives of seriously ill patients.

Feedback:
The first important thing to note about this activity is that most of the objectives cannot be satisfactorily assessed using only one method. Nursing performance is multi-dimensional and requires a variety of methods to adequately assess competence.

Assessing knowledge
For convenience we will consider the knowledge components of the objectives first. Knowledge is an important component of clinical performance and assessment of knowledge is a necessary but not sufficient step in the assessment of competence.

For recognition of myocardial infarction students would need to be able to list the clinical features of myocardial infarction or describe the typical appearance of a patient with myocardial infarction. There are a number of methods you could have chosen to assess this objective. Most commonly used methods would be:

1.   Short answer questions
Short answer questions would be appropriate here because the answer you are expecting could be easily covered in a few lines and would be easy to mark. The student's score could be based on the number of diagnostic features stated correctly in the answer. An example of a short answer question would be:

> List five clinical features which would
> lead you to suspect that a patient has
> suffered a myocardial infarction,
> or,
> Describe the typical clinical presentation
> of a patient who is suffering an acute
> myocardial infarction.

Short answer questions are a convenient way to
test **recall** of information because they are quick
to complete and to mark and therefore allow you to
set a large number of questions which sample a
broad area of knowledge. Their disadvantage is that
they encourage students to learn lists of facts
which are easily and quickly recalled, rather than
to learn underlying principles and to develop the
habit of thinking things through.

2.   Multiple choice questions (MCQ)
MCQ could be appropriate here because the question
is factual and requires little explanation by the
student. There are a number of different types of
MCQ (see Anderson, 1981 and Kirby, 1982 for
examples), but the most common and easiest to mark
is the one from five, so called because the student
is required to choose one correct response from
five possible alternatives. An example of this type
of MCQ is:

> A fifty five year old man is brought to the
> emergency clinic with the story that he has
> collapsed in the street. He is pale, sweaty,
> has a weak, rapid irregular pulse, and is
> breathless. Among his personal effects is a
> bottle of glyceryl trinitrate tablets. The
> most likely cause of his collapse is:
>
> a)   asthma
> b)   ruptured aorta
> c)   acute myocardial infarction
> d)   stroke
> e)   pneumonia

Actually it is very hard to write a good MCQ
item for an objective such as this because it is
difficult to find sufficient distractors (incorrect
alternatives) which are realistic enough to test
the students' knowledge. The above MCQ is likely to

201

be a very easy one which is answered correctly by almost all of the students.

Another commonly used MCQ is the true/false type:

Acute myocardial infarction:
a)	is always accompanied by chest pain	T	F
b)	may give rise to arrhythmias	T	F
c)	gives rise to symptoms of shock	T	F
d)	causes T wave inversion on ECG	T	F
e)	is fatal in 70% of cases	T	F

Once again such items are difficult to write because there are few absolutes in medicine. Only a very naive student would agree with a question which includes the words 'always' or 'never'. Sometimes performance in MCQ tests is an assessment of how 'test-wise' the students are rather than how much they know.

The advantages of MCQ are that they are fast to answer, fast to mark, and are reasonably objective, that is they do not rely on individual judgements by examiners but have a predetermined set of correct answers which can be marked by computer if necessary. These advantages are balanced, however, by the fact that good MCQs (those which are not ambiguous, or not too easy or not too hard, or don't give too many clues or too few realistic alternatives) are very time-consuming to develop. For this reason teachers often keep a bank of MCQs which have been shown to be good ones and which are used from year to year. The development of good MCQ items and tests, the analysis of item performance and the interpretation of student performance is a complex process which involves statistical manipulation. If you intend to use MCQ examinations you would be well-advised to consult with your local educational testing service or to refer to the many detailed texts available (for example, Ebel, 1972; Adkins 1974; Cox & Ewan, 1982, Chs 37,38,39).

The disadvantage of MCQs is that they provide all of the information and students need only to **recognise** the correct information. Recognition requires even less thinking than recall and it encourages students to learn patterns of symptoms and lists of facts which can be learned at a glance. MCQs can be written to test problem solving skills by, for example, providing a case history in the stem and a sequence of items which require students to make progressive steps towards solution of the clinical problem (see Joorabchi, 1981 & Kirby, 1982). However, there are probably better ways to assess problem-solving skills and some of these will be dealt with later in this chapter.

3.   Essay questions
Essay questions are less appropriate for a purely factual response because they are difficult and quite time-consuming to mark. For testing factual knowledge, essay questions have no advantage over a series of short answer questions.

4.   Oral examinations
Oral examinations are an extremely inefficient and ineffective way to test students' factual knowledge. They are time-consuming and they are not standardised so that different students may be asked questions in different ways and their responses judged according to the impressions of the examiner rather than some predetermined criteria established by the teacher. In addition many students find oral examinations very stressful and fail to perform well even though they may know quite a lot of factual material.

What we have said about the knowledge component of objective (i) also applies to the knowledge component of objective (iv) - students could be asked to list the items on the cardiac arrest trolley in a short answer question or to identify the correct items in a multiple choice question. Similarly basic knowledge required in history taking could be assessed by asking the student to write a list of the questions she would ask, or in objective (v) to write a brief description of the role of the nurse in the management of a cardiac arrest, or to choose the most appropriate options from a multiple choice series of alternatives in response to a specific scenario in the question stem. However, objectives (ii), (iv) and (v) imply much more than simple knowledge, they also imply that the student will apply that knowledge to the various nursing responsibilities. It is not sufficient to ascertain that students know what should be done, it is important to make sure that they actually do what needs to be done at the appropriate times, in a manner which is consistent with good nursing care.

Assessing clinical performance

For recording a history and assessing the nursing needs of a patient the student would have to demonstrate the ability to actually produce the history and assessment. The only real way to assess this is to either observe the student taking a history or to examine the written history and assessment which the student provides after spending time with the patient. The written product of the interview will tell you whether the student has obtained all the relevant information and been able to synthesise it in a meaningful way to formulate an assessment of nursing care needs, but it will tell you nothing about the spirit of the encounter or how well the student managed to establish rapport and develop a relationship with the patient. Direct observation or interview of the patient is an additional component which would have to be added to the assessment to provide information about the students' mastery of those relationship (or affective) objectives. We will leave consideration of the assessment of affective objectives for the moment and concentrate on assessment of skill performance.

Direct observation of skill performance can be arranged in a number of ways:

1.   Formal clinical examinations
Clinical examinations can be set up and arrangements made for real patients from the wards or clinics to be present. Students may be left alone with the patient for a while, or the examiners may stay to observe all of the students' performance. Facilities permitting, a desirable alternative could be to have examiners observing through a one way window or on closed circuit TV.

Of course it would be necessary for both student and patient to know that they were being observed but the lack of the actual physical presence of the examiner would probably enhance the interaction.

2. Assessment in training

It might be more appropriate for certain skills to be assessed during the course of the students' clinical training. In-service assessment is appropriate for skills which are difficult to set up for a formal examination, such as assisting with a lumbar puncture, or skills which carry an element of risk and require close supervision, or just day to day skills and procedures such as lifting patients, presenting ward reports etc. which need to be assessed but which are not necessarily part of summative assessment. Assessment in training has been discussed earlier in this chapter when it was emphasised that the distinction should be drawn between assessment to learn and assessment to certify.

3. Simulations

In some situations it is not desirable to assess students' performance with real patients or in real situations because of risk or discomfort or because the situation is not suited to examination conditions. Morgan, Luke and Henry (1979) have described videotaped interactions and written case studies as simulations intended to assess students' ability to assess nursing care needs. Simulations also give you more control over what happens in the assessment. For example, for the present objective different students may receive very different patients to interview and the amount of information they are able to elicit may not be entirely due to their skill in history taking. Similarly some patients might present more straightforward problems than others and might be easier to assess. This is unavoidable because it would be unreasonable to expect the same patient to submit to several interviews by several different students. An alternative is to train simulated patients to provide a standard history, or for the examiner or teacher to play the role of the patient and provide the history. This latter method raises some problems if only one examiner is present because it is difficult to be both interviewee and examiner at the same time.

205

<u>Observation Tools</u> - The two most commonly used tools for performance assessment in all of these contexts are checklists and rating scales:

<u>Checklists</u> require the observer to judge whether certain behaviour has taken place. They are most effective where components of performance can be specified in detail (Katz & Snow, 1980). Checklists provide a list of detailed behaviours within a performance, sometimes in the sequence in which they should occur, and the observer is asked to record whether the behaviour was observed or not observed. A third option such as 'not applicable' should be included. Because checklists are so detailed they provide a useful profile of performance which can be discussed with the student. If any essential component of the performance is omitted the student can be said not to have achieved mastery on that criterion and should be required to present for further assessment after more practice. Common important errors made by students should also be included so that the observer can note errors of commission as well as errors of omission. An example of a checklist for assessing students' ability to administer intramuscular medications is provided in table 7.1. Alternative examples can be found in De Mers (1978), Schneider (1979) and Katz & Snow (1980).

As the checklist demonstrates, it is possible to include considerations of attitudes and relationship skills in checklists for the observation of skill performance. Stecchi et al. (1983) have gone one step further in devising a clinical evaluation tool in the form of a checklist which can be applied in a variety of settings. They describe the tool as being

'organised around 22 objectives which define the areas of clinical and theoretical competence the student is expected to achieve by the end of the junior year. To the right of each objective are four columns corresponding to the four clinical nursing courses. Each course column is subdivided into two additional columns designated 'S' for satisfactory and 'U' for unsatisfactory.

TABLE 7.2 :
   CHECKLIST: Administration of intramuscular
                 injection

Activities:	Observed	Not observed	N/A
1. Checks medication as required by law	( )	( )	( )
2. Measures the ordered dose	( )	( )	( )
3. Checks patient identification	( )	( )	( )
4. Assembles appropriate sterile needle and syringe	( )	( )	( )
5. Aspirates sterile medication	( )	( )	( )
6. Prepares appropriate site	( )	( )	( )
7. Inserts sterile needle at 90 degrees	( )	( )	( )
8. Withdraws plunger (removes needle if blood appears)	( )	( )	( )
9. Injects the total dose	( )	( )	( )

Behaviour guides:	Yes	No	N/A
a) Approaches patient with confidence and courtesy	( )	( )	( )
b) Explains in a way the patient can understand	( )	( )	( )
c) Anticipates patient's need for privacy	( )	( )	( )
d) Fails to make allowances for individual differences in pain tolerance	( )	( )	( )
e) Notices cues indicating discomfort and attempts to alleviate it	( )	( )	( )
f) Focuses attention on the procedure to exclusion of all else	( )	( )	( )

TABLE 7.3 :

RATING SCALE : Ward Management Skills

Key: 7 - Excellent
     6 - Above average
     5 - Average
     4 - Below average
     3 - Poor
     2 - Unsatisfactory
     1 - Insufficient information available

Record keeping: Consider   7 6 5 4 3 2 1
legibility, accuracy, detail,
systematic presentation.

Relationships with patients &   7 6 5 4 3 2 1
  relatives:
Consider sensitivity to needs,
giving clear & appropriate
information, caring approach

Relationship with other   7 6 5 4 3 2 1
  professionals:
Consider collaboration, giving
clear/courteous instructions,
accepting constructive criticism

Reliability/dependability: 7 6 5 4 3 2 1
Consider doing what is expected
and required, organisation of
tasks, reaction under stress.

One copy of the tool is kept in the clinical unit and follows the student to the next clinical unit, another copy is for student self-evaluation and a third copy is kept on record for faculty evaluation. The article includes a copy of the checklist.

Rating scales require judgements by the observer about how well the performance meets the set criteria. Rating scales usually provide from 3 to 7 options for the observer to quantify the level of performance of the student in comparison with an ideal standard. It is therefore important that the observers use a common standard. Some inexperienced observers make the mistake of rating a student nurse's performance against the standard they would expect of a graduate or experienced nurse. Assessors should spend time together identifying the standard to be used. A further problem with rating scales is that since they provide a means for quantifying the observer's judgements they provide a false sense of security. Numerical scores derived from rating scales can be just as subjective as unstructured opinions unless observers are trained to provide reliable (that is reproducible) judgements. Combining ratings from different observers can help to eliminate observer bias or unreliability. Rating scales are most appropriate to assess traits such as efficiency, judgement, ability to work with others (Irby & Dohner, 1976), and the ability to adapt to local characteristics and variations (Katz & Snow, 1980, p. 32). Further examples of rating scales can be found in the references cited above under checklists. One example of a rating scale is given in table 7.2, but the variety of formats possible is considerable.

Remember that observers will need to be trained in the use of any rating scale that you choose or develop, and that baseline criteria for making the judgements should be explicit.

Two other methods which have been used to assess clinical performance of nurses are the anecdotal record and the critical incident technique.

209

The anecdotal record suffers from the fact that it is anecdotal and that the information recorded is likely to be unsystematic, may be unrepresentative of the student's behaviour in general and difficult to interpret for assessment purposes. The anecdotal record is often a mix of fact and opinion. Rines (1963) has suggested a standard format for recording anecdotal information which attempts to differentiate between fact and opinion - the anecdotal record should consist of three segments, a description of the context of the event, a description of the actual behaviour witnessed and only then a statement of the observer's opinion of the behaviour. Even when this approach is employed however, there is difficulty in obtaining balance and spread of observations in relation to the objectives, and the information gathered is unlikely to be reliable enough for use in normative assessment, although it can be a useful approach to identifying students' problems in the formative context.

The critical incident technique assumes that raters will make inferences about a person's general competence on the basis of the person's performance in a number of specific situations (Sims, 1976). In order that the data is generalisable a number of general headings under which performance is to be assessed by grouping similar incidents must be established. In this way critical incidents can be used to develop a performance record based on core behaviours (Fivars & Gosnell, 1966). This approach fits well with criterion-referenced assessment where the core behaviours for mastery have been identified. Unfortunately there are logistic problems which limit the usefulness of the technique, principally arising from uneven enthusiasm, interest and commitment among clinical staff who are expected to be reporters, and from the difficulties in establishing consensus on categories into which incidents fit. Dachelet et al (1981) used critical incidents to obtain a holistic perspective, a broad picture of activities in a clinical practicum setting - they provide details of the categories and criteria used to classify incidents. Sims (1976) reported that nursing sisters disliked the technique because of the connotations of the term 'critical'. Flanagan

(1954) specified criteria for the use of critical incidents to assess clinical performance:

1. The actual behaviour must be reported rather than general traits.
2. The behaviour must be actually observed by the reporter.
3. All relevant factors in the situation must be given.
4. The observer/reporter must make a definite judgement of the 'criticalness' of the behaviour.
5. The observer/reporter must make it clear why the behaviour is considered to be critical.

An example of a simple format for recording critical incidents is the following:

TABLE 7.4 : CRITICAL INCIDENT REPORT

Name of student:
Name of reporter:

Think of the last time you observed this student nurse do something that you thought was especially effective in contributing to patient care.

What led up to the situation?

Exactly what did the nurse do?

Why do you feel it was particularly effective?

Trained observers can provide valuable data on performance using the critical incident technique and it can also be extended as a method for student self-reports where students are asked to identify critical incidents in their learning experience, and areas in which they need more assistance. Stainton (1983) has developed an alternative to critical incident recording which fits more easily with ward routine. A Clinical Experience Record for each student is kept in a loose leaf binder in the ward and includes the following information:

A. Assignment - details of the patient
B. Learning Experience - including reasons why the particular assignment was chosen for the student, and the preparation necessary before undertaking the assignment.
C. Nursing care planning - anecdotal notations and evidence of preparation done for the assignment.
D. Comments regarding implementation - notations of how the student carries out the plan. Behavioural descriptions are recorded as objectively as possible.

The record provides a composite picture of experiences offered and allows progress to be reviewed with the learner.

Activity:
In the light of what we have said so far perhaps you would like to reconsider the rest of the objectives in the activity on page 199 What methods would you use to assess the objectives remaining?

iii) Students must be able to develop a nursing plan for the care of a patient admitted to the coronary car unit.

iv) Students must be able to correctly set up the cardiac arrest trolley.

v) Students must be able to assist in the emergency management of a patient with cardiac arrest.

vi) Students must demonstrate care and concern for the wellbeing of patients in their care and consideration for the needs of the relatives of seriously ill patients.

Feedback:
<u>Developing a nursing plan</u> could be assessed effectively by the critical incident or anecdotal record techniques or by the use of simulated patient encounters or even paper and pencil computerised simulations. Development of simulations for both learning and assessment have been discussed in Chapter 6, and a most comprehensive review of the construction and use of written simulations can be found in McGuire, Solomon & Bashook (1976). Specific examples of assessments of medical students' problem solving skills which can be readily adapted for nursing students are provided by McGuire (1980a & b). The Nursing Undergraduate Review for Self Evaluation (Kirby, 1982) also contains numerous examples of sequential multiple choice questions which require students to assess a patient history and develop appropriate nursing responses.

Essay questions have been widely used to assess problem-solving skills but often the questions are not specific enough and students have to guess what the examiner wants them to write about. In addition essays are difficult to mark consistently - two different examiners may give quite different marks for the same essay unless they have agreed on some specific marking scheme which includes a list of the major points which should be covered in the essay. For this objective however a better method would be the modified essay question or MEQ (Knox, 1980). Modified essay questions are a series of short answer questions which are related to a single clinical problem and which proceed from an initial scenario of the problem to its sequential development, progressively providing more information and requesting decisions from the student. Since subsequent questions sometimes provide the answers to previous questions special measures must be taken in administering the test, for example each page can be collected as the student finishes it and the next step in the problem given to the student. An advantage of the MEQ is that even if the student answers a question wrongly, she does not necessarily lose marks for the whole MEQ. She can redeem herself in the next section by realising her error and progessing down the correct path. Marking the MEQ is also more reliable because

213

essential points in each section can be defined as
criteria. Discussion of the MEQ after the
examination can be a learning experience which
helps the students to develop a systematic approach
to discussion of a clinical problem.

Setting up a cardiac arrest trolley is an excellent
example of a performance which would be most
effectively assessed by the use of a checklist
since it consists of a well-defined set of
observable behaviours which are easily specified
and require little independent judgement by the
observer.

Assisting in the emergency management of a patient
with cardiac arrest could theoretically be assessed
by observation in the real setting using a rating
scale or critical incident format, but in practice
it is very unlikely that such behaviours would be
amenable to observation. The most feasible approach
to assessing this very important objective is to
assess theoretical knowledge in a written
examination and to assess ability to apply that
information in a realistic simulation in the
nursing laboratory, where checklists, rating scales
or other clinical performance observation schedules
can be used to both assess and provide feedback to
students on performance.

Demonstrating care and concern for patients and
relatives is, of course, an attitudinal or
affective objective which can only be assessed by
direct observation of the student over a broad
range of time and clinical experiences. Anecdotal
records, critical incidents and rating scales all
lend themselves to the assessment of affective
objectives. There are a number of methods available
for written assessments of attitudes such as
semantic differential scales, questionnaires, self
reports (Girod, 1973; Oppenheim, 1966); Weinholtz &
Stritter, 1982) and for simulated assessments such
as responding to videotaped vignettes of events or
people. These methods however suffer from problems
of validity in that they demonstrate whether
students know what the desired or appropriate
attitudes are but they do not demonstrate that the
student actually behaves according to those
attitudes in the real situation. They are open to

'fakability' and to biases imposed by students providing socially acceptable responses.

There is always a value position inherent in attitudinal objectives and criteria and some teachers feel uncomfortable in asserting particular values or providing feedback to students whose values are not consonant with their own. Nevertheless values are an integral part of nursing and must be taken into account in learning and assessment. Reilly (1978, p. 63) clarifies the problem somewhat with the following statement : 'When students are asked for opinions, feelings, beliefs or points of view on value related issues, the opinion cannot be graded. However, the logic, accuracy and completeness of the rationale for the opinion can be graded.' For example, students can be given a problem to solve which requires a choice on a value related issue and their responses judged on their ability to identify alternatives, predict consequences and provide a rationale for the preferred action. Essays would be an appropriate assessment method for this type of objective.

Attitudes, perhaps more than any other type of learning, require formative rather than summative assessment, and sensitive feedback where deficiencies are identified. Gordon (1978) has proposed a clinical model for assessment of student affect which recognises this sensitivity. The basic components of the model are:

1. Statement of affective objectives - begin with a general statement of the attitude and develop a narrative statement of a situation in which this attitude would be demonstrated.

2. Screen for potential behaviour problems to provide an early warning system.

3. Clarify problems - involve the student and encourage self-assessment.

4. Assess specific behaviours and clarify whether differences from criterion are due to value differences or perception differences between student and advisor.

5. Provide assistance - joint planning, specific commitments to tasks.

215

6.   Determine the potential seriousness of the problem.

7.   If the problem has not responded to the above, formally inspect performance with due notice to the student.

8.   Take administrative action to suspend or dismiss if the student does not respond to the above measures and counselling.

Improving   reliability   of   clinical   performance assessment.
      All of these methods of assessing clinical performance experience problems in reliability derived from the fact that the examiner is required to make a judgement about the student's performance. Clinical examiners may differ in the standards they set, thus a single student may receive two quite different marks from two different examiners who are using different criteria to judge competence. Thus observation of performance may not be a reliable way to assign marks or grades unless preventive measures are taken.

      Activity:
      Suggest ways in which the reliability of assessment of clinical performance can be improved.

Feedback:
      This question has exercised the minds of nurse educators more than any other issue in assessment (see Rines, 1963; Woolley, 1977; Schneider, 1979). Basically, reliability can be improved by achieving consensus on specific unambiguous criteria, by making those criteria known to examiners, by incorporating the criteria into assessment tools, by testing and training examiners to use those tools, by basing assessments on a sample of student behaviour rather than a single episode and by checking on the statistical profile of assessment marks.
      Consensus on criteria can only be achieved by involving assessors or examiners in the development

216

of learning objectives and assessment tools, pre-assessment conferences can be used to achieve consensus where necessary, to discuss criteria with new teachers or assessors and to train assessors in the use of the assessment tools. After the assessments have been completed **statistical profiles** of student perfomance and examiner performance can be used to identify atypical or isolated performance difficulties of students and characteristic marking behaviours of assessors - some mark consistently high and some consistently low. Armed with this information you can make more reliable judgements about overall student performance, you can alter the weight given to certain assessments and you can plan future teams of assessors who balance each other or may be able to influence each other to more closely approach the norm of marking practice.

CHARACTERISTICS OF A GOOD ASSESSMENT

Deciding on the purposes of assessment and the types of assessment most suited to the learning objectives are only part of the assessment task. Making your chosen assessment methods good ones is also very important.

What is a good assessment?

Activity:
Based on your experience and what you have read in this chapter so far list the characteristics of a good assessment.

A good assessment is valid
An assessment is said to be valid if it tests what it is supposed to test. Assessments should test important skills, knowledge and attitudes which are the objectives of the course.

For example, an essay test used to assess a student's ability to perform a procedure is not a valid test. It tests only what the student knows should be. done, but does not test whether the student is actually able to do it. A valid test of this skill would be the actual performance, under real or simulated conditions, of the procedure.

A good assessment is comprehensive

The assessment should test achievement of the essential objectives of the course and a wide and representative range of the other objectives of the course. Many assessments test only the students' memory for facts. A good test will require students to apply facts to the solution of problems or the discussion of important issues, or the performance of manual skills. Higher level objectives should be adequately represented among assessment criteria. This means that a variety of assessment methods must be used.

A good assessment is fair

All students must have an equal chance to perform well if they have learned well. Examination items should be specific and unambiguous so that there is no risk that some students might give a wrong answer because they have mistaken the meaning of the question. If possible, tests should be spread over a period of time so that students who are having an 'off day' for some reason or another have an opportunity to be assessed under more favourable circumstances. In assessments of clinical performance steps should be taken to provide for a variety of assessments and assessors to avoid errors due to bias of observers or other extraneous factors.

Marking schemes for questions such as MCQs should be developed so that students who know the right answer score more, on average, than students who are just guessing.

A good assessment is reliable

You must be able to rely on the consistency and accuracy of scores given. Reliability of assessors can be tested by asking two different examiners to assess the same student on achievement of the same objectives, or by asking the same examiner to assess the same test at two different times. If the scores are similar or the same then the assessment is reliable. Loustau et al. (1980), using videotapes to establish rater reliability for assessing clinical performance found that cognitive items were more difficult to reach agreement on than skill items. Training sessions using videotaped student-patient interactions improved the reliability of raters using a clinical evaluation tool.

Assessments using MCQs and MEQs are very reliable because there is one agreed answer and examiners do not have to exercise judgement in giving scores. MCQs are frequently marked by computers. Unfortunately, while these exams are very reliable they are not valid for a wide range of objectives in nursing.

Essay questions, oral examinations, examination of student products such as assignments, nursing reports and projects, and direct observation of clinical performance, while being more valid assessments of nursing objectives are frequently not very reliable because they require examiners to exercise their judgement and opinions about student performance. Reliability of these types of assessment can be improved by:

a) training examiners in the application of standard criteria to establish inter-rater reliability
b) providing standard checklists or rating scales which make criteria explicit
c) averaging the scores given by more than one examiner.

A good assessment is economical

Assessments should be economical in time as well as money. Essays are very time-consuming to mark but do not take long to set whereas MCQs are quick to mark but their development is time-consuming. Clinical observation schedules which are lengthy and not feasible within normal ward routines have very little chance of being used as they are intended or of providing valid and reliable results.

A good assessment can be used to help students learn

Assessments should, wherever possible be a learning experience for students. In informal assessment students can be encouraged to develop skills in peer and self-assessment. In formal assessment for certification or mastery students should be informed of criteria used to make judgements and of their personal performance in relation to those criteria. Formative assessment should be an integral part of learning and students should always have access to an advisor with whom they can discuss their achievements and their

219

deficiencies.

A good assessment can give you information about the success of your course

Assessments should be regarded by you as a research tool to help you identify patterns in your students' performance which may indicate problems with curriculum, prerequisites, and objectives and implementation of your course.

Levine (1978) has summarised these and more detailed considerations in selecting evaluation instruments.

SUMMARY

Students learn what they need to learn in order to pass exams. This is a fact of life. Assessments must therefore test what students must learn in order to be competent nurses. You will not be able to measure or assess all levels of learning if you use only one or a few types of assessment method. A variety of assessment methods will help you to assess a broader range of the knowledge, skills and attitudes that your students must demonstrate in order to be competent nurses.

If the assessment results are unsatisfactory, or the pass rate is low, or if significant numbers of students are not achieving mastery in a reasonable time, use the assessment results as a guide to problem areas in your course. Assessment should be a tool for improving both teaching and learning.

Chapter 8.

EVALUATING TEACHING

Just as assessment of student performance is a necessary component of helping students learn to be better nurses, so is assessment of teaching a necessary component of helping you and your teaching colleagues to offer better courses.

When you have completed this chapter you should be able to plan a program of evaluation to assist you in improving the courses that you offer.

CRITERIA FOR EVALUATION

Activity:
Consider the course that you teach. After working through this book you have decided to try some new approaches to that course but you would like to be able to determine whether they are effective. What criteria will you use to evaluate your new course?

Feedback:
Possibly the first criterion you chose to evaluate the success of your new course was students' performance in the examinations. This is as far as many teachers go in trying to determine the value of their course, but this is not far enough. You cannot be sure that student performance is totally dependent on your teaching or your course. Many other factors are also involved. For example, students may already have known a great deal of what you thought you were teaching them; or

they may not have performed well because they did not have sufficient background knowledge to benefit fully from your course. Or, perhaps your course is taught at the same time as another more demanding course which takes most of the students' study efforts; or perhaps your students are so highly motivated that they will perform well regardless of the quality of the course you offer. For all of these reasons and more, student examination performance is only one of many criteria you could use in evaluating your course.

The following table is a summary of the criteria you might use to evaluate courses.

TABLE 8.1 : CRITERIA FOR COURSE EVALUATION

General criteria	**Specific criteria**
Effectiveness	Achievement of course objectives.
	Retention of learning to be used in subsequent courses.
	On-the-job performance.
	Occurrence of unexpected outcomes (good or bad).
Acceptability	Appropriateness of objectives.
	Satisfaction with resources and teaching methods.
	Learning environment & climate.
	Appropriateness of assessment methods.
Feasibility	Time spent in course preparation.
	Class hours and private study time required by students.
	Ease of availability of resources.
	Cost of resources (time or money).
	Availability of appropriate facilities.
	Interrelatedness with other courses - is there interference with timetables, assignments, exams etc?

Of course, it may not be possible or even appropriate to use all of these criteria but they are included here to give you some idea of the options from which you can choose.

Choice of criteria

Activity:
How would you choose which criteria to include in your evaluation?

Feedback:
The answer to this question depends entirely on your circumstances and the reasons why you have chosen to evaluate. For example, if budgetary restrictions are a problem for you, you may place a high priority on evaluating resources and teaching methods to determine whether expenditure is cost-effective. If, on the other hand, you have indications that students have not been performing satisfactorily in certain areas of subsequent courses you may choose to evaluate achievement of course objectives or even the appropriateness of those objectives. **The rule of thumb is to begin your evaluation in an area in which either a problem has been identified, or in which a decision has to be made** (with regard to use of resources for example).

Choosing criteria is only part of the problem, once you have decided where you wish to start you must then decide how you will collect information to help you make decisions about those criteria.

SOURCES OF INFORMATION

Activity:
Refer to the list of criteria in the feedback to the first activity in this chapter and construct a table which indicates sources of information for each criterion.

Feedback:

Specific criteria	Sources of information
Achievement of objectives	Pre- & post-test student performance.
Retention of learning	Feedback from teachers of other courses.
On-the-job performance	Direct observation. Feedback from clinical supervisors Feedback from patients. Feedback from recent graduates on their preparation for the job.
Unexpected outcomes	Observations of classroom process. Interview with students.
Appropriateness of objectives	'Expert opinion'. Feedback from other teachers. Information about on-the-job performance.
Resources & Teaching methods	Teacher opinion based on observations in class. Student opinion (questionnaire or discussion). Peer observation.
Learning environment & climate	Teacher opinion. Student opinion. Peer observation.
Appropriateness of assessment	Review of assessment to ensure that it reflects objectives. Profile & analysis of student performance.
Time spent in course preparation.	Teacher's observations.

Class hours & study time	Student diaries.
Availability of resources	Teacher's observations. Student feedback.
Cost of resources	Teacher's observations. Administrative records.
Availability of facilities	Teacher's observations. Student feedback.
Interrelatedness with other courses	Feedback from, and negotiation with other teachers.

You can see that a **comprehensive evaluation involves collection of information from a variety of sources.** It may not be appropriate or feasible to gather information from all or even most of them but the following guidelines will assist you in deciding how you wish to use some of the most important sources of feedback on your course.

Student performance

Student performance is an important source of information for course evaluation, although as we mentioned earlier it is not necessarily the most important source since it provides only part of the information you need to have. Deficiencies in student performance can indicate that there is a problem, they might even indicate in which component of the course the problem lies but they will rarely be able to tell you exactly what is the cause of the problem. Failure to achieve some of the course objectives will be revealed on item analysis of a well-constructed assessment however you will need to use other sources of information to determine whether the students failed to achieve the objectives because they lacked relevant prerequisite learning, whether the teaching in that area was insufficient or ineffective, whether the resources were appropriate, whether there was some extraneous variable affecting student learning at the time or whether the assessment actually reflected the objectives.

Teacher's observations

You will notice that you, as the teacher are an important source of information for evaluating the course. You will be aware, every time you teach, of aspects of your classes which were particularly successful and aspects which you would do differently next time. Course evaluation by direct observation requires that you take note of these experiences and use them to improve your subsequent teaching.

Student opinion

Students are also an important source of information for course evaluation. Teachers sometimes object to asking for feedback from students because they fear that students are not qualified to judge or that they will be unfair in their criticism. The experience of teachers who do use student feedback as a source of information is that students, when offered some responsibility are happy to take a responsible approach. It is also important however, to demonstrate that student feedback has been considered and, where appropriate, used for course revision otherwise students quickly become cynical and rightly so. It is important to ask student opinion only in areas in which you are prepared to accept their judgement. For example students might not be competent to judge whether you have presented your subject matter accurately but they are competent to judge whether you have presented it clearly or whether the resources you have recommended helped their understanding.

For some purposes, where the class is large or where you feel anonymous feedback will more accurately reflect student opinion you may choose to use a student opinion questionnaire. For other purposes it may be more appropriate to talk personally with students individually or as a class to gain feedback on general or specific aspects of their experiences in your classes and other components of the course. The personal approach is appropriate in situations where a personal relationship already exists, as between student and clinical supervisor, and is particularly useful for maximising the value of individual student experiences since it allows a two way interaction and the opportunity for clarification of specific problems.

If circumstances call for a questionnaire the same principles apply as to any form of questionnaire design - decide what information you want, determine whether a free response or rating scale would give you the most useful information, write the questions and pilot test the instrument before administering it to the students. Useful advice on the development of instruments for student evaluation of teaching can be found in Centra (1980).

Student opinion is probably most appropriately sought in a context in which it provides private feedback to the teacher concerned. Use of student feedback for administrative decision-making such as promotion is a sensitive area and one which should be fully explored and discussed with teachers to ensure its appropriate and effective use without destruction of morale.

Peer observation

Another major source of information is your teaching colleagues, or if your school has an educational development unit, you may wish to ask the staff of that unit to provide a professional appraisal of your course design, your resources or your teaching performance.

Understandably many teachers have no wish to expose their weaknesses to their colleagues and therefore many opportunities are missed for teachers to help each other to improve the courses they teach. This state of affairs has not been helped by the practice, in some schools, of conducting formal evaluations of teaching for administrative purposes such as salary grading or promotion. A purely administrative approach to teacher evaluation can be counterproductive because, although it rewards teaching accomplishments it tends to generate a climate of threat which is not conducive to development of teaching skills for personal satisfaction, or for the benefit of the students. Evaluation of teaching which emphasises personal development and job satisfaction rather than administrative rewards should generate a more positive learning environment within the school. An approach which stresses mutual cooperation among teachers will be more helpful than one in which teachers are encouraged to criticise each other's efforts.

Discussing course changes and plans and eliciting comments from other teachers helps an atmosphere of openness to develop. This is particularly relevant if your course is likely to affect students' study habits and therefore spill over onto other courses. For example, adoption of a mastery-based approach will have implications for timetabling in other courses to avoid clashes of assessment periods. Checking whether this has happened and whether problems or benefits have been created for other teachers should be part of your course evaluation. Remember, your courses do not occur in isolation and therefore should not be evaluated in isolation, but in the context of their relationship to other courses and the overall objectives of the program. Anatomy classes must prepare students for what they will need to do in safely administering intra-muscular injections. If they do not, then they are not effective, no matter how well the students have performed in the Anatomy examination.

Unintended outcomes

Don't forget, that even though you have defined objectives and assessed your students' achievement of those objectives and evaluated your course partially on how well students have achieved the objectives, other outcomes of learning which were not planned might occur. Sometimes these will be desirable outcomes and sometimes they will not be, however if you are not alert to the possibility of unintended outcomes you will not identify them and will miss opportunities for improving your course.

REPORTING EVALUATION DATA

This chapter assumes that you are evaluating your course mainly for your own benefit and for the benefit of your students. A more detailed treatment of evaluation for the purpose of improvement can be found in Rotem & Abbatt (1982) and Dressell (1980). Other reasons for evaluation would be for research purposes, to prove the superiority or cost-effectiveness of some teaching approach, or for administrative purposes to allow official decisions to be made about administrative actions such as curriculum review or teacher promotion. Consideration of both of those purposes is beyond the scope of this book, however details of evaluation for administrative decision-making can be found in Roe & McDonald (1983) and Joint Committee on Standards for Educational Evaluation (1981).

To the extent that your course forms part of a larger educational program you have a responsibility to share the results of evaluation with colleagues. This is perhaps not as important in areas such as personal evaluation of teaching performance but it is very important in areas which indicate the effectiveness of particular teaching or assessment methods, the appropriateness of course objectives and the readiness of students to learn certain aspects of the course and to use certain resources and facilities. In addition, since you have probably involved colleagues and students in providing you with information and feedback it is important that you demonstrate that their efforts were worthwhile by discussing proposed actions with them and indicating how their feedback assisted you to make the decisions you have taken.

The way you communicate the results of your evaluation efforts will depend on your particular situation, some teachers choose to publish in the professional literature to gain a wider audience, some offer in-house seminars or establish regular review meetings of interested teachers, and some choose informal discussions over a cup of coffee. Whichever your preference remember that feedback on teaching is most effective when it is framed constructively, when it offers specific indicators for improvement and when it is supported by concrete examples rather than abstract ideals. Don't be overly concerned if some of your information is derived from subjective opinions – these are the best indicators of learning environment, an important aspect of nursing education. 'Anthropological' approaches to evaluation have been shown to be as effective as experimental approaches in providing feedback to teachers which they are prepared to accept (Schermerhorn & Williams, 1979). In addition observational, even anecdotal data may be more valid in the evaluation of much of nursing education than is an attempt to experimentally prove that 'Method A' is better than 'Method B'. The literature abounds with such research-oriented evaluations which are almost always confounded by the multitude of uncontrollable variables occurring in any educational program.

Evaluation of teaching should be an ongoing part of every teacher's teaching and learning program. Information may be sought formally or informally, verbally or through questionnaires or course documents, or it may be serendipitously collected along the way as critical incidents or unexpected outcomes make themselves apparent. Whatever the source of the information it should be evaluated for its potential contribution to better student learning and, where possible and desirable, changes should be implemented and evaluated in their turn.

SUMMARY

Activity:
Develop a plan for conducting an evaluation of your course.

Feedback:
Use the following checklist to ensure that you have included the necessary steps in your course evaluation plan.

CHECKLIST FOR COURSE EVALUATION

1. Why do you wish to carry out an evaluation - is the purpose for improvement, for research or for administrative reasons?

2. What questions will you ask to provide you with information suited to your purposes?

3. What sources of information will you use?

4. What instruments or resources will you need for the acquisition of that information?

5. How will you analyse and use the data you gather?

6. What are the factors in the context or climate of your school which will determine the way you report your evaluation results?

7. What methods will you use for reporting the results of your evaluation which you have decided to make public?

8. How will you plan to implement changes which are indicated by your evaluation - consider the context of your course?

9. How will you evaluate the changes you have made?

We hope that this book will have helped you to both evaluate your teaching efforts and plan appropriate educational responses to what you learn about your program. Teaching and learning is a dynamic process, healthy educational programs, like children, are those which continue to develop. Your ability and willingness to adapt to changing needs and contexts will serve as a valuable model for the flexibility your students will need as professionals practising in a rapidly changing environment.

REFERENCES

Abbatt, F.R. (1980) Teaching for Better Learning. A guide for teachers of primary health care staff, WHO, Geneva.

Abercrombie, M.L.J. (1979) Aims and Techniques of Group Teaching, Society for Research into Higher Education, London.

Acker, S., Megarry, J., Nisbet, S. & Hoyle, E. (1984) Women and Education , World Yearbook of Education, Kogan Page, London.

Adam, E. (1983) Frontiers of nursing in the 21st century: development of models and theories on the concept of nursing, J. Advanced Nursing, 8, 41-45.

Adkins, D.C. (1974) Test Construction, 2nd Edition, Charles E. Merrill Publ. Co. Columbus, Ohio.

Alexander, M. (1982) Integrating theory and practice: An experiment evaluated, in Henderson, M.S. (ed.) Nursing Education, Churchill Livingstone, Edinburgh.

Allen, M. (1977) Evaluation of Educational Programmes in Nursing, WHO, Geneva.

Anderson, B. (1976) Basic Nurse Education Curriculum. A Research Report submitted to the Commission of Advanced Education by Cumberland College of Health Sciences, Sydney.

Anderson, J. (1981) The MCQ Controversy - A Review, Medical Teacher, 3, 150-6.

Andrews, S. & Hutchinson, S. (1981) Teaching nursing ethics: A practical approach, J. Nursing Educ., 20, 6-11.

Applbaum, R.L., Bodaken, E.M., Sereno, K.K. & Anatol, K.W.E. (1974) The Process of Group

References

Communication, Science Research Associates Inc., Chicago.

Aroskar, M. (1980) Anatomy of an ethical dilemma, Am. J. Nursing, 80, 658-63.

Ausubel, D.P. (1960) Use of Advance Organizers in the Learning & Retention of Meaningful Verbal Material, J. Educ. Psychol., 51, 267-72.

Barrows, H.S. (1971) Simulated Patients, Charles C. Thomas, Chicago.

Barrows, H.S. & Tamblyn, R.M. (1980) Problem-based Learning. An Approach to Medical Education, Springer Services on Medical Education, Springer Publ. Co., New York.

Baumann, A. & Bourbonnais, F. (1982) Nursing decision-making in critical care areas, J. Advanced Nursing, 7, 435-46.

Bennett, M. (1976) A two-paradigm approach to the study of the decision processes of nurses in relation to clinical judgement. Unpublished Honours thesis, Monash University, Melbourne.

Benoliel, J.Q. (1983) Ethics in nursing practice and education, Nursing Outlook, 31, 211-15.

Bevis, E. (1973) Curriculum Building in Nursing: A process, C.V. Mosby & Co., St. Louis.

Blank, M. & Solomon, F. (1969) How shall the disadvantaged be taught? Child Development, 40, 47-61.

Bligh, D.A. (1972) What's the Use of Lectures? Penguin Books, Harmondsworth.

Block, J.H. (1971) Introduction to Mastery Learning: Theory and Practice, Ch.1 in Block, J.H. (ed.) Mastery Learning:Theory and Practice, Holt, Rinehart & Winston, New York.

Bloom, B.S. (1971) Mastery Learning, in Block, J.H. (ed.) op. cit.

Boud, D. & Pearson, M. (1979) The trigger film: A stimulus for affective learning, Programmed Learning & Educational Technology, 16, 52-6.

Brewer, A. (1983) Nurses, Nursing and New Technology: Implications of a Dynamic Technological Environment, Australian Studies in Health Service Administration No.47, School of Health Administration, University of New South Wales, Sydney.

Brown, G. (1978) Lecturing and Explaining, Methuen, London.

Brown, G. & Tomlinson, D. (1980) How to Improve Handouts, Medical Teacher, 2, 215-20.

233

Rekerences

Brown, J.D. Lewis, R.B. & Harcleroad, F.F. (1973) AV Instruction Technology Media and Methods, 5th Edition, McGraw Hill, New York.

Bruner, J.S., Goodnow, J.J. & Austin, G.A. (1956) A Study of Thinking, J. Wiley & Sons, New York.

Bruner, J.S. (1962) On Knowing, Harvard University Press, Cambridge, Massachusetts.

Campbell, A.V. (1975) Moral Dilemmas in Medicine, Churchill Livingstone, Edinburgh.

Carlson, C. (1970) Behavioural Concepts and Nursing Intervention, J.B. Lippincott, Philadelphia.

Carper, B.A. (1978) Fundamental patterns of knowing in nursing, Annals of Advances in Nursing Science, 1, 13-23.

Celebreeze, A.J. (1966) The Technological Revolution and Education, as quoted in Brewer, A. op. cit.

Centra, P.L. (1980) Determining Faculty Effectiveness, Jossey-Bass Publ., San Francisco.

Chakrabaty, E. (1983) Research in Nursing: School of Nursing Libraries as Information Resources for Nurse Education, in Davis, B.D. Research into Nurse Education, Croom Helm, London.

Chapman, C.M. (1980) The rights and responsibilities of nurses and patients, J. Advanced Nursing, 5, 127-34.

-      (1983) The paradigm of nursing, J. Advanced Nursing, 8, 269-72.

Chinn, P. & Jacobs, M. (1983) Theory and Nursing. A Systematic Approach, C.V. Mosby & Co., St. Louis.

Clark, J. (1982) Development of models and theories on the concept of nursing, J. Advanced Nursing, 7, 129-34.

Colliere, M-F. (1980) Development of primary health care, Int. Nurs. Rev., 27, 169-72.

Conley, V.C. (1973) Curriculum and Instruction in Nursing, Little Brown & Co., Boston.

Coombe, E.I., Jabbusch, B.J., Jones, M.C., Pesznecker, B.L., Ruff, C.M. & Young, K.J. (1981) An incremental approach to self-directed learning, J. Nursing Educ., 20, 30-35.

Cowart, M.E. & Allen, R.F. (1982) Moral development of health care professionals begins with sensitizing: 33 sample encounters, J. Nursing Educ., 21, 4-7.

References

Cox, K.R. & Ewan, C.E. (1982) The Medical Teacher, Churchill-Livingstone, Edinburgh.

Craig, S.L. (1980) Theory development and its relevance for nursing, J. Advanced Nursing, 5, 349-55.

Creighton, H., Hart, G. & Clear, W. (1983) An Analysis of Patient Care Provided by Nursing Personnel, Nurse's Education Board of New South Wales, Sydney.

Cronbach, L.J. & Snow, R.E. (1977) Aptitudes and Instructional Methods, Irvington Publ. Inc. New York.

Crow, R. (1982) Frontiers of nursing: the twenty first century: development of models and theories on the concept of nursing, J. Advanced Nursing, 7, 111-16.

Curtin, L. (1978) Nursing ethics: Theories and pragmatics, Nursing Forum, 17, 4-11.

- (1978) A proposed model for critical analysis, Nursing Forum, 17, 12-17.

Cyrs, T.E. (1976) Managing students through the use of learning modules, J. Pract. Nursing, 20, 32-35.

Dachelet, C.Z., Wemett, M.F, Garling, E.J., Craig-Kuhn, K., Kent, N. & Kitzman, H.J. (1981) The critical incident technique applied to the evaluation of the clinical practicum setting, J. Nursing Educ., 20, 15-31.

Davis, A.J. (1979) Ethics rounds with intensive care nurses, Nursing Clinics of North America, 14, 45-55.

Davis, A. & Aroskar, M. (1978) Ethical Dilemmas and Nursing Practice, Appleton-Century-Crofts, New York.

Davis, A. & Krueger, J. (eds.) (1980) Patients, Nurses and Ethics, American Journal of Nursing Co., New York.

Davis, B.D. (ed.) (1983) Research into Nurse Education, Croom Helm, London.

De Mers, J.L. (1978) Observational Assessment of Performance, Ch. 8 in Morgan, M.K. & Irby, D.M. Evaluating Clinical Competence in the Health Professions, C.V. Mosby & Co., St. Louis.

de Tornyay, R. (1971) Strategies for Teaching Nursing, John Wiley & Sons, New York.

Dewey, J. (1917) Democracy and Education, MacMillan, New York.

References

Donaldson, S.K. (1983) Let us not abandon the humanities, Nursing Outlook, 31, 40-3.

Donaldson, S.K. & Crowley, D.M. (1978) The discipline of nursing, Nursing Outlook, 26, 113-20.

Draugsvold, N. (1982) Assessing and assisting the adult learner: a model, in Jenkins, E., King, B. & Gray, G. Issues in Australian Nursing, Churchill Livingstone, Edinburgh.

Dressel, P.L. (1980) Improving Degree Programs, Jossey-Bass Publ., San Francisco.

Durbridge, N. & Gale, J. (1980) How to use prepared TV material and films in medical education, Medical Teacher, 2, 163-67.

Eastman Kodak, (1980) The Joy of Photography, Addison-Wesley Publ. Co., Rochester, New York.

Ebel, R.L. (1972) Essentials of Educational Measurement, 2nd Edition, Prentice-Hall Inc. Englewood Cliffs, New Jersey.

Engel, C.E. (1980) For the use of objectives, Medical Teacher, 2, 232-37.

Ewan, C.E. (1981) How to prepare and use slides, Medical Teacher, 3, 52-62.

- (ed.) (1982) Self-Instruction: A Strategy for Education of Health Personnel, Review Paper No. 1, Centre for Medical Education Research & Development, University of New South Wales, Sydney.

Fawcett, J. (1978) The 'what' of theory development, pp. 17-33 in National League for Nursing Theory Development: What, Why, How?, NLN, New York.

- (1980) On research and the professionalization of nursing, Nursing Forum, 19, 310-17.

Fenner, K. (1980) Ethics and Law in Nursing: Professional Perspectives, D. Van Nostrand, New York.

Fishel, A.H. & Johnson, G.A. (1981) The three-way conference - nursing student, nursing supervisor and nursing educator, J. Nursing Educ., 20, 18-23.

Fivars, G. & Gosnell, D. (1976) Nursing Evaluation: The Problem and the Process. The Critical Incident Technique, MacMillan Co. New York.

Flanagan, J.C. (1954) The Critical Incident Technique, Psychol. Bull., 51, 327-58.

Flaskerud, J.H. (1983) Utilizing a nursing conceptual model in basic level curriculum development, J. Nursing Educ., 22, 224-27.

References

Foley, R.P. & Smilansky, J. (1980) Teaching Techniques. A Handbook for Health Professions, McGraw Hill, New York.

Freire, P. (1970) Pedagogy of the Oppressed, Seabury Press, New York.

Gagne, R.M. (1976) Essentials of Learning for Instruction, Dryden Press, Hinsdale, Illinois.

Garfield, E. (1980) Portable information - is the dream becoming a reality? Current Contents, 16, 5-12.

Garrick, C.E. (1978) Design of instructional illustrations in Medicine, J. Audiovisual Media in Medicine, 1, 161-73.

Geach, B. (1974) The problem-solving technique: is it relevant to practice? The Canadian Nurse, January, pp.21-22.

Gibson, S. (1980) A critique of the objectives model of curriculum design applied to the education and training of district nurses, J. Advanced Nursing, 5, 161-67.

Girod, G.R. (1973) Writing and Assessing Attitudinal Objectives, Charles E. Merrill Publ. Co., Columbus, Ohio.

Gordon, M.J. (1978) Assessment of Student Affect: A Clinical Approach, Ch.7 in Morgan, M.K. & Irby, D.M. op.cit.

Guest-Lee, S. (1979) Television in Medicine, Part 1: Choosing a television system, J. Audiovisual Media in Medicine, 2, 64-66.

- (1979) Television in Medicine, Part 2: Planning and preparation for small team television production, J. Audiovisual Media in Medicine, 2, 118-21.

Hartley, J. (1978) Designing Instructional Text, Kogan Page, London.

Hartley, J. & Davies, I.K. (1978) Notetaking: A critical review, Programmed Learning & Educational Technology, 15, 207-24.

Heath, J. (1982) Curriculum Design in Nursing. A practical guide for course planners, NHS Learning Resources Unit, Sheffield.

Heath, J. & Marson, S. (1979) Its a taxing process, Nursing Mirror, August 23, pp.75-78.

Helmer, O. (1967) Analysis of the Future. The Delphi Technique, RAND Corporation, Santa Monica.

Henderson, M. (ed.) (1982) Nursing Education, Churchill Livingstone, Edinburgh.

Henderson, V. (1966) The Nature of Nursing, MacMillan, New York.

Heywood, J. (1982) Pitfalls and Planning in Student Teaching, Kogan Page, London.

Hill, M., Gortner, S.R. & Scott, J. (1980) Educational research in nursing - an overview, Int. Nurs. Rev., 3, 10-17.

Hinchliff, S.M. (ed.) (1979) Teaching Clinical Nursing, Churchill-Livingstone, Edinburgh.

Holzemer, W.L. (1982) Research in nursing education, J. Nursing Educ., 21, No.8, whole issue.

Hope, J. & McAra, P. (1983) Games Nurses Play, Pergamon Press, Sydney.

Hudson, L. (1968) Frames of Mind: Ability, Perception and Self-Perception in the Arts and Sciences, Methuen, London.

Hunt, D.R. (1982) Patient Management Problems for Teaching and Assessment, in Cox, K.R. & Ewan, C.E. op. cit.

Hynes, K. (1980) An ethical decision system, in Davis, A. & Krueger, J. (eds.), op. cit.

Illich, I. (1971) Deschooling Society, Harper & Row, New York.

Infante, M.S. (1975) The Clinical Laboratory in Nursing Education, John Wiley & Sons, New York.

-      (1978) Meeting Program Objectives in the Clinical Laboratory, in National League for Nursing, Utilization of the Clinical Laboratory in Baccalaureate Nursing Programs, NLN, New York.

Irby, D.M. & Dohner, C.W. (1976) Student Clinical Performance, Ch.20 in Ford, C.W. & Morgan, M.K. (eds.) Teaching in the Health Professions, C.V. Mosby & Co., St. Louis.

Jerrett, M.D. & Ross, M. (1982) Learning to nurse: the family as the unit of care, J. Advanced Nursing, 7, 461-68.

Johnson, D.N. & Johnson, R.T. (1974) Instructional goal structure: Cooperative, competitive or individualistic? Rev. Educ. Res., 44, 213-41.

Johnston, M. (1979) Toward a culture of caring: children, their environment and change, MCN, 4, 210-14.

Joint Committee on Standards for Educational Evaluation, (1981) Standards for Evaluation of Educational Programs, Projects and Materials, McGraw Hill, New York.

References

Joorabchi, B. (1981) How to construct problem-solving MCQs, Medical Teacher, 3, 9-13.

Kagan, J. (1965) Impulsive & Reflective Children: Significance of Conceptual Tempo in Learning in the Educational Process, Rand McNally, Chicago.

Kagan, N. (1980) Influencing human interaction - Eighteen years with IPR, in Hess, K. (ed.) Psychotherapy Supervision: Theory, Research & Practice, John Wiley & Sons, New York.

Kamenka, E. & Tay, A. (1981) Human Rights and the Australian Tradition in Tay, A. (ed.) Teaching Human Rights, An Australian Symposium, UNESCO, Australian Govt. Printing Service, Canberra.

Katz, F.M. & Snow, R.E. (1980) Assessing Health Workers' Performance. A Manual for Training and Supervision, Public Health Papers No. 72, WHO, Geneva.

Kerr, F.F. (ed.) (1976) Changing the Curriculum, Unibooks, London.

Kilmon, C., Powell, P. & Whitman, N. (1980) Clinical objectives for nurse practitioner students, J. Nursing Educ., 18, 37-41.

Kirby, S. (1977) Testing: For what purpose? Norm-referencing or Criterion-referencing, The Lamp, August, 27-29.

- (ed.) (1982) Nursing Undergraduate Review for Self Education, Adis Health Science Press, Sydney.

Kirchoff, K. & Holzemer, W. (1979) Student learning and a computer-assisted instructional program, Nurse Educator, 18, 22-30.

Knowles, M. (1975) Self-Directed Learning - A guide for learners and teachers, Association Press, Follett Publ., Chicago.

Knox, J.D.E. (1980) How to use modified essay questions, Medical Teacher, 2, 20-24.

Kochman, R.F. (1976) Are letter grades and modularized nursing programs compatible? J. Nursing Educ., 15, 25-27.

Kodak Pamphlet No. S-22 Effective Lecture Slides, Eastman Kodak Co. Rochester, New York.

Kodak Pamphlet No. S-24 Legibility: Artwork to Screen, Eastman Kodak Co. Rochester, New York.

Kohlberg, L. (1972) The cognitive-developmental approach to moral education, The Humanist, 32, 12-18.

Krumme, U.S. (1975) The case for criterion-referenced measurement, <u>Nursing Outlook</u>, <u>23</u>, 764-79.

Kruse, L.C. & Fagerbarger, D.M. (1982) Development and implementation of a contract grading system, <u>J. Nursing Educ.</u>, <u>21</u>, 31-37.

Laduca, A. (1975) Professional performance situation model for health professions education: occupational therapy, as quoted in McGaghie, W.C., Miller, G., Sajid, A. & Telder, T., <u>Competency-based Curriculum Development in Medical Education: An Introduction</u>, WHO, Geneva.

Lamb, M. (1982) Nursing ethics and nursing education: past perspectives and recent developments, in Henderson, M., <u>op. cit.</u>

Lawrence, S.A. & Rena, M. (1983) Curriculum development, philosophy, objectives and conceptual framework, <u>Nursing Outlook</u>, <u>31</u>, 160-63.

Lee, A. (1978a) Small group teaching in Microbiology 1. Objectives, <u>Med. J. Aust.</u>, <u>1</u>, 487-99.

-    (1978b) Small group teaching in Microbiology 2. Techniques, <u>Med. J. Aust.</u>, <u>1</u>, 551-54.

-    (1978c) Small group teaching in Microbiology 3. Examples, <u>Med. J. Aust.</u>, <u>1</u>, 605-7.

-    (1978d) Small group teaching in Microbiology 4. Comments and revision, <u>Med. J. Aust.</u>, <u>1</u>, 645-47.

Lesser, G. (1972) Pedagogical adaptations to individual differences: some research findings, in Sperry, G.H. (ed.) <u>Learning Performance in Individual Differences</u>, Scott Foresman, Illinois.

Levine, H. (1978) Selecting Evaluation Instruments, Ch4 in Morgan, H.K. & Irby, D.M., <u>op. cit.</u>

Levine, M. (1977) Nursing ethics and the ethical nurse, <u>Am. J. Nursing</u>, <u>77</u>, 845-49.

-    (1980) The ethics of computer technology in health care, <u>Nursing Forum</u>, <u>19</u>, 193-98.

Loustau, A., Lentz, M., Lee, K., McKenna, M., Hirako, S., Fontaine Walker, W. & Wyman Goldsmith, J. (1980) Evaluating students' clinical performance: Using videotape to establish rater reliability, <u>J. Nursing Educ.</u>, <u>19</u>, 10-17.

Lovell, R.B. (1980) <u>Adult Learning</u>, Croom Helm, London.

Re6erences

McCloskey, J. (1981) The professionalisation of nursing. United States and England, Int. Nurs. Rev., 28, 40-47.

McElhinney, T.K. (1983) Placing the humanities perspective in the health professional curriculum, J. Allied Health, 12, 221-28.

McGuire, C.H., Solomon, L.M. & Bashook, P.G. (1976) Construction and Use of Written Simulations, Psychological Corp., New York.

McGuire, C.H. (1980a) Assessment of problem-solving skills, 1, Medical Teacher, 2, 74-79.

-       (1980b) Assessment of problem-solving skills, 2, Medical Teacher, 2, 118-22.

McLeish, J., Matheson, W. & Park, J. (1973) The Psychology of the Learning Group, Hutchison & Co., London.

Marson, S. (1979) Objectives: Markers along the way, Nursing Mirror, August 16, pp.72-74.

Maslow, A.H. (1943) A theory of human motivation, Psychol. Rev., 50, 370-96.

Matejski, M. (1982) Ethical issues in the health care system, J. Allied Health, 11, 131-39.

Megarry, J. (1979) Developments in Simulation & Gaming in Howe, A. & Romiszowski, A.J. (eds.) International Yearbook of Educational and Instructional Technology, Kogan Page, London.

Meleis, A.I. & Burton, P.S. (1981) Innovative educational changes: a paradigm, Int. J. Nursing Studies, 18, 33-39.

Melia, K.M. (1982) 'Tell it as it is' - a qualitative methodology and nursing research: understanding the student's world, J. Advanced Nursing, 7, 327-35.

Messick, S. (ed.) (1976) Individuality in Learning: Implications of Cognitive Styles and Creativity for Human Development, Jossey-Bass Publ., San Francisco.

Miller, Sister P. (1975) Clinical knowledge: A needed curriculum emphasis, Nursing Outlook, 23, 222-24.

Mitchell, J.J. (1981) The use of case studies in Bioethics courses, J. Nursing Educ., 20, 31-36.

Morgan, B., Luke, C. & Herbert, J. (1979) Evaluating clinical proficiency, Nursing Outlook, 27, 540-44.

Morgan, M.K. & Irby, D.M. (1978) Evaluating Clinical Competence in the Health Professions, C.V.

Mosby & Co., St Louis.

Morse, J.M. (1983) An ethnoscientific analysis of comfort: A preliminary investigation, Nursing Papers, 15, 6-19.

Munhall, P. (1982) Moral development: A prerequisite, J. Nursing Educ., 21, 11-15.

Norris, C.M. (1975) Restlessness: A nursing phenomenon in search of meaning, Nursing Outlook, 23, 103-107.

Novak, J.D. (1979) Improvement of laboratory teaching, The American Biology Teacher, 41, 467-70.

- (1980) Handbook for Learning How to Learn Program, Cornell University, New York.

O'Brien, P. (1978) The Delphi Technique. A review of research, South Australian J. Educ. Res., 1, 57-75.

Oppenhiem, A.N. (1966) Questionnaire Design and Attitude Measurement, Basic Books, New York.

O'Rourke, K. (1983) Moral development considerations in nursing curricula, J. Nursing Educ., 22, 108-13.

Orton, H. (ed.) (1983) Ward learning climate and student response, in Davis, B.D. (ed.) Research into Nurse Education, Croom Helm, London.

Pascasio, A. (1975) Clinical facilities, in Ford, C.W. & Morgan, M.K. (eds.) op. cit.

Pashuk, G. (1983) Catalogue of Educational Films, Tertiary Education Research Centre, University of New South Wales, Sydney.

Pask, G. (1976) Styles and strategies of learning, Brit. J. of Educ. Psychol., 46, 128-48.

Pence, T. (1983) Ethics in Nursing. An annotated bibliography, NLN Publ. No. 201936, New York.

Phenix, P.H. (1966) Realms of Meaning, McGraw Hill, New York.

Piaget, J. (1971) Science of Education and the Psychology of the Child, Longman, London.

Powell, L.S. (1973) Lecturing, Pitman, London.

Purtilo, R.B. (1983) Ethics in allied health education: State of the art, J. Allied Health, 12, 210-20.

Quinn, F.M. (1980) The Principles and Practice of Nurse Education, Croom Helm, London.

Rabb, J.D. (1976) Implications of moral and ethical issues for nurses, Nursing Forum, 15, 168-79.

References

Raths, L.E. (1966) <u>Values and Teaching</u>, Charles E. Merrill Publ. Co., Columbus, Ohio. (as quoted in Reilly, D.E., Teaching and Evaluating the Affective Domain in Nursing Progrms).

Reilly, D.E. (ed.) (1978) <u>Teaching and Evaluating the Affective Domain in Nursing Programs</u>, Charles B. Slack, Detroit.

- (1980) <u>Behavioural Objectives in Evaluation in Nursing</u>, Appleton-Century-Crofts, New York.

Reynolds, W. & Cormack, D. (1982) Clinical teaching: an evaluation of a problem-oriented approach to psychiatric nurse education, <u>J. Advanced Nursing</u>, 7, 231-37.

Rines, A.R. (1963) <u>Evaluating Student Progress in Learning the Practice of Nursing</u>, Teachers College Press, Columbus University.

Robertson, C.M. (1980) <u>Clinical Teaching</u>, Pitman Medical, London.

Rogers, C. (1969) <u>Freedom to Learn</u>, Charles E. Merrill Publ. Co., Columbus, Ohio.

Roe, E. & McDonald, R. (1983) <u>Informed Professional Judgement: A Handbook for Evaluation in Higher Education</u>, University of Queensland Press, St. Lucia.

Romanell, P. (1977) Ethics, moral conflicts and choice, <u>Am. J. Nursing</u>, 77, 850-55.

Romiszowski, A.J. (1981) <u>Designing Instructional Systems</u>, Kogan Page, London.

Roper, M. (1980) <u>The Elements of Nursing</u>, Churchill Livingstone, Edinburgh.

Rotem, A. & Abbatt, F.R. (1982) <u>Self-assessment for Teachers of Health Workers</u>, WHO, Geneva.

Rule, J. (1978) The professional ethic in nursing, <u>J. Advanced Nursing</u>, 3, 3-8.

Ryan-Merritt, M. (1982) A teaching strategy for evaluating assertive behaviour change, <u>J. Nursing Educ.</u>, 21, 13-16.

Schermerhorn, G.R. & Williams, R.G. (1979) An empirical comparison of responsive and pre-ordinate approaches to program evaluation, <u>Educational Evaluation & Policy Analysis</u>, 1, 55-60.

Schneider, H.L. (1979) <u>Evaluation of Nursing Competence</u>, Little, Brown & Co., Boston.

Schoolcraft, V. & Delaney, C. (1982) Contract grading in clinical evaluation, <u>J. Nursing Educ.</u>, 21, 6-14.

References

Schramm, W. (ed.) (1972) Quality in Instructional Television, University Press of Hawaii, Honolulu.

Schweer, J.E. (1972) Creative Teaching in Clinical Nursing, C.V. Mosby & Co., St. Louis.

Schwirian, P. (1981) Toward an explanatory model of nursing performance, Nursing Res., 30, 247-53.

Simon , S., Howe, L. & Kirschenbaum, H. (1978) Values Clarification. A Handbook of Practical Strategies for Teachers and Students, A & W Publishers, New York.

Simpson, I.H. (1979) From Student to Nurse, Cambridge University Press, Cambridge.

Simpson, M.H. (1980) Objections to objectives, Medical Teacher, 2, 229-31.

Sims, A. (1976) The critical incident technique in evaluating student nurse performance, Int. J. Nursing Studies, 13, 123-30.

Singer, P. (1981) Teaching Human Rights, in Tay, A. (ed.) Teaching Human Rights, An Australian Symposium, UNESCO, Canberra.

Smallegan, M.J. (1982) Teaching through groups, J. Nursing Educ., 21, 23-31.

Smith, L. (1982) Models of nursing as the basis for curriculum development: some rationales and implications, J. Advanced Nursing, 7, 117-27.

Srinivasan, L. (1977) Perspectives on Non-formal Adult Learning, World Education, New York.

Stainton, M.C. (1982) The birth of nursing science, Canadian Nurse, November, pp.24-28.

- (1983) A format for recording the clinical performance of nursing students, J. Nursing Educ., 22, 114-6.

Stecchi, J.M., Woltman, S.J., Wall-Haas, C., Heggestad, B. & Zier, M. (1983) Comprehensive approach to clinical evaluation: One teaching team's solution to clinical evaluation of students in multiple settings, J. Nursing Educ., 22, 38-46.

Stenhouse, L. (1975) An Introduction to Curriculum Research and Development, Heineman, London.

Stevens, B.J. (1979) Nursing Theory. Analysis, Application, Evaluation, Little Brown, & Co. Boston.

Sullivan, E. & Brye, C. (1983) Nursing's future: Use of the Delphi Technique for curriculum planning, J. Nursing Educ., 22, 187-89.

244

Swanson, E.A. & Dalsing, C.W. (1980) Independent study: A curriculum expander, J. Nursing Educ., 19, 11-15.

Sweeney, M.A., O'Malley, M. & Freeman, E. (1982) Development of a computer simulation to evaluate the clinical performance of nursing students, J. Nursing Educ., 21, 28-38.

Taba, H. (1962) Curriculum Development Theory and Practice, Harcourt, Brace & World, New York.

Taylor, S., Brodish, M. & Brown, H. (1979) Creative learning experience for student nurses, J. Nursing Educ., 18, 16-18.

Tindall, K., Collins, B. & Reid, D. (1973) The Electric Classroom. Audio Visual Methods in Teaching, McGraw Hill, Sydney.

Toffler, A. (1981) The Third Wave, Pan Books, London.

Turney, C., Cairns, L.G., Eltis, K.J., Hatton, N., Thew, D.M., Powler, J. & Wright, R. (1983) Supervisor Development Programmes Role Handbook, University of Sydney Press, Sydney.

Uustal, D. (1977) The use of values clarification in nursing practice, J. Cont. Educ. Nursing, 8, 8-13.

Warwick, D. (1973) Curriculum Structure and Design, Unibooks, London.

Watson, C.R.R. (1982) Colour microfiche in biomedical education, Ch.31 in Cox, K.R. & Ewan, C.E. op. cit.

Weatherston, L. (1979) Theory of nursing: creating effective care, J. Advanced Nursing, 4, 365-75.

Weinholtz, D. & Stritter, F. (1982) How to plan an assessment of students' attitudes, Medical Teacher, 4, 95-101.

WHO Division of Health Manpower Development (1976) Facilitating Teaching-Learning with Modules: An Approach for Nurse Midwife Teachers, British Life Assurance Trust, Centre for Health & Medical Education, London.

Wilson, J.D. (1981) Student Learning in Higher Education, Croom Helm, London.

Wilson-Barnett, J. (1983) Nursing Research. Ten Studies in Patient Care, John Wiley & Sons, Chichester.

Witkin, H.A. et al. (1954) Personality through Perception, Harper & Row, New York.

Witkin, H.A., Moore, C.A., Goodenough, D.R. & Cox, P.W. (1977) Field dependent and field independent cognitive styles and their educational implications, Rev. Educ. Res., 47, 1-64.

Wong, J. (1979) The inability to transfer classroom learning to clinical nursing practice: A learning problem and its remedial plan, J. Res. Nursing, 4, 161-68.

Woolley, A.S. (1977) The long and tortured history of clinical evaluation, Nursing Outlook, 25, 308-15.

Yura, H. & Walsh, M.B. (1978) The Nursing Process, 3rd Edition, Appleton-Century-Crofts, New York.

INDEX

13. 74 -

13